CONTENTS

Bear in mind that:

THIS WORKING GUIDE IS ABOUT
PROBLEMS THAT THE PHW MAY FACE
DURING DAILY WORK.

THE PROBLEMS, THE TEXT AND THE
DRAWINGS SHOULD BE **ADAPTED**
TO THE CONDITIONS OF EACH COUNTRY
AND EACH COMMUNITY IN WHICH THE
GUIDE IS TO BE USED.

★

INTRODUCTION

Only a few countries have succeeded in ensuring a wide coverage of their population by health care services. Although successful country schemes vary in many respects, they have some features in common. Thus, in each country or area, the government started by forming, reinforcing or recognizing a local community organization and treated it as a "partner" in the enterprise. This partner had five functions. It laid down priorities; it organized community action for problems that could not be resolved by individuals; it controlled the primary health care service by selecting, appointing or "legitimizing" the primary health worker; it assisted in financing services and/or in sharing the labour involved; and it linked health action with broader community goals.*

Another feature common to successful schemes is that their systems of primary health care either were linked with the indigenous system or had built into them some social qualities from the old system. In this sense the new did not destroy the old but built upon it, and the link between the old and the new was a socially relevant change. Furthermore, they were politically oriented to the equitable distribution of welfare among the masses, and health development was viewed as part of community development.

Another common element is the use of a primary health worker who is not necessarily a member of the usual health service staff, i.e. a doctor or a nurse. This person is frequently a villager selected by the community and trained locally (in some cases for as little as two to four months initially). He or she can be an unpaid volunteer, or partially or totally supported by the official health services or by the village people in cash or kind, with responsibilities for promoting health and preventing and treating disease.

---

* Newell, K.W., ed., Health by the people, Geneva. World Health Organization, 1975, p.193.

This kind of community health scheme must, of course, have government approval and support. The government promotes it by legislation, training, supervision, referral facilities, funds, stocks and means of supply. One of the government's main duties is to organize suitable training of its health workers at various levels of health care delivery, and to provide on-the-job technical guidance and continuing learning opportunities.

This working guide outlines the structure and content of training for the primary health worker on the basis of the most common health problems of communities in developing countries.

Part I can be used by the primary health worker as a learning text and also as a guide in his work. Part II is addressed to the health workers' teachers, tutors and supervisors. Part III discusses the adaptation of the book to local conditions; this can be done only in the country where it is to be used.

Before drafting learning material, there are several prerequisites which should be met. Task analysis has to be carried out and job descriptions written. These must be preceded by an analysis that includes specific country ecology, health conditions, and existing health service systems and possibilities. The present document is an illustration of what can be done; the WHO Working Group who prepared it took, as a basis, some general assumptions about problems and conditions common to many areas of developing countries with similar socioeconomic conditions. It was assumed also that the purpose was to satisfy minimal needs for community health and social well-being with modest resources in places insufficiently covered by a health infrastructure, official or private.

This working document, therefore, is not specific for any country and must be adapted for use in any particular country in accordance with its own needs, structures and potentialities.

The Primary Health Worker (PHW) profile

Who is the PHW?

The PHW is a man or woman who can read and write, and is selected by the local community or with their agreement to deal with the health problems of individuals and the community.

Conditions of work

The PHW will be responsible both to the local community authorities and to a supervisor appointed by the official health services. He will follow his supervisor's instructions and work with him in a team.

The PHW will be paid for his work, in cash or in kind, by the local community; he may be full-time or part-time, depending on requirements.

The local community will provide a hut or a room to be used only for his health work.

What training will the PHW receive?

The PHW will receive initial training for six to eight weeks from the official health service of the country. Training will be practical and given near his home. Preferably, the supervisor should give much of the instruction and be responsible for continued on-the-spot or cyclical training. A plan for this further training should be worked out.

What will the PHW do?

The work of the PHW will cover both health care and community development, as man's health and that of the community is very much influenced by any improvement in the environment.

The health work of the PHW will be restricted to what he has learned. The PHW must realize his limitations and know that there is only a restricted number of things he can do. He will not be able to solve all the problems he meets, but he should be able to deal with the most common and urgent.

The community development work of the PHW should serve to encourage the local authorities and the people to show initiative and take an interest in any activity likely to improve their living conditions. He should always consider what can be done locally with the community's own resources at the least possible cost.

The PHW's duties will depend on the problems he meets. These will vary from one country to another; it is impossible to draw up a list of problems valid throughout the world.

It is assumed, however, that some problems and concerns are common to all countries. This assumption has led the WHO Working Group who prepared this Guide to select the problems included in Part I on the basis of the following criteria:

- frequency of disease

- demand from the public

- danger to the individual

- danger to the community

- technical feasibility of action for a PHW

- economic consequences of the "problem".

From the problems selected, which make up Part I of the present document, one can outline the functions of a PHW:

1. Care for the sick, protect the health of the people and look after community hygiene.

2. Give care and advice to anyone who consults him, in accordance with the instructions contained in this Guide or given by his supervisor.

3.   Send patients to the nearest health centre or hospital (evacuation or referral) in any case in which the Guide instructs him to do so and in any case not covered by the Guide. The PHW should, therefore, confine his care and treatment to those cases, conditions and situations described in the Guide.

4.   With the authorization of the local authorities, visit all dwellings and advise the people how to prevent disease and learn good habits of hygiene.

5.   Make regular reports to the local authorities on the health of the people and on conditions of hygiene in the community. Get from the local authorities and the people the support he needs for his work.

6.   Keep as close contact as possible with his supervisor so as to be able to give of his best in his work and to obtain the equipment and supplies he needs.

7.   Promote community development activities and play an active part in them.

      To discharge these functions the PHW:

      a)   is available at all times to respond to any emergency calls

      b)   acts in all circumstances with common-sense and devotion to duty, and is aware of his limitations and responsibilities

      c)   does not leave the community without first informing the local authorities

      d)   takes part in the training organized by the health service.

      The PHW should spend some time with other social/developmental workers concerned with improving agricultural practices, food protection, water supply, house economics, etc. He must know about services and opportunities for development available in his district and keep his community well informed.

      It follows then that the PHW is the practical expression of a community's determination to be responsible for its own health care and to make up for any deficiencies that might exist in the health service coverage. The PHW should improve the community's participation in what will be part of a provincial/national health project planned and run by the national health authorities with the active contribution of the people.

★

Bear in mind that:

SEVERAL PHWs MAY WORK AS A TEAM IN THE SAME VILLAGE WITH THEIR SUPERVISOR.

CERTAIN PROBLEMS MAY BE SOLVED AND CERTAIN TASKS MAY BE CARRIED OUT BY A MALE PHW AND OTHERS BY A FEMALE PHW, DEPENDING ON THE WISHES OF THE COMMUNITY, ITS HABITS AND ITS MEANS.

★

PART I

★

Working Guide

★ ★ ★

Bear in mind that:

A PRIMARY HEALTH WORKER (PHW) DOES NOT PRACTISE IN ISOLATION. HE SHOULD BE A PART OF A HEALTH SYSTEM AND AS SUCH BE REGULARLY SUPERVISED. HE SHOULD KNOW WHERE AND WHEN TO SEEK GUIDANCE AND TO REFER PATIENTS WHO ARE SERIOUSLY ILL OR WHOSE ILLNESS IS BEYOND HIS COMPETENCE TO TREAT.

★

This Working Guide, when adapted to local conditions, is primarily intended for PHWs, who will use it first during their training and then as a reference book while working. Obviously, the trainers and supervisors of PHWs also have to be very familiar with it so that their advice, guidance and instructions can be easily understood and correspond with what has been previously learned by the PHWs.

It covers thirty-four problems which are considered to be the most common and therefore the most likely to be found in any given rural community. Only thirty-three problems have been detailed, since Problem 1.1 "Vaccination" has only been mentioned as a reminder; it should be considered in the context of national programmes. The thirty-four problems have been grouped under seven main headings:

1. Communicable diseases

2. Maternal care

3. Child health. Nutrition

4. Accidents

5. Village and home sanitation

6. Other common problems

7. Community development

Each problem begins with a few words of explanation; this is followed by a special page of "learning objectives", i.e. what the PHW should know and be able to do after he has studied the problem. In each case, preventive measures are suggested and simple treatment indicated, when possible; otherwise referral to the health centre or hospital is necessary.

Annex 1 gives the list of medicines used in this Working Guide, how they should be administered, and the doses according to age. It is extremely important to review this list and to adapt it to local usage.

In Annex 2 a few techniques are described, namely, how to take the temperature, intramuscular and subcutaneous injections, and bandaging. Other techniques are given under specific problems, such as how to clean a wound, or build a stretcher; they are listed on page 268.

The anatomical diagrams in Annex 3 may facilitate the work of the trainers of PHWs when they answer questions on human anatomy or physiology.

VACCINATION

When germs attack the body, we catch diseases which make us feverish. A vaccine is a substance which is made from the germs that cause diseases and which can fight these germs in the body.

To prevent some of the diseases caused by germs, healthy people are given vaccines by injection (polio vaccine is given by mouth); this is called vaccination.*

If it is decided to vaccinate the inhabitants of your community, you will be informed by your supervisor, who will give you the necessary instructions.

This problem is not discussed further in this book because you will follow the directions laid down by the vaccination programmes of the country where you work.

---

* TO CURE people who are already ill, other drugs (such as penicillin, chloroquine and sulfadiazine) are given which kill the germs that have already entered the body or prevent them from multiplying.

FEVER

A PATIENT HAS A FEVER WHEN HIS TEMPERATURE IS OVER 37.5^{o}C.

A CHILD UNDER SCHOOL AGE WHOSE TEMPERATURE IS OVER 38°C MAY BE VERY ILL. ALWAYS GIVE HIM ASPIRIN IN ADDITION TO THE TREATMENT FOR HIS ILLNESS, AND TELL HIS MOTHER TO GIVE HIM A LOT OF LIQUIDS TO DRINK, BECAUSE FEVER, LIKE DIARRHOEA, MAKES THE PATIENT LOSE A LOT OF WATER.

FEVER

LEARNING OBJECTIVES

At the end of his training, the PHW should be able to:

1. Decide if a patient has a fever:
    1.1. take the temperature
    1.2. read a thermometer

2. Identify three signs that show that a patient has a fever

3. Treat a patient who has a fever but no other signs

4. List five conditions where the patient with a fever must be sent to the hospital or health centre

5. Send to the hospital or health centre a feverish patient with any of those five conditions

FEVER

A PERSON BECOMES FEVERISH

when the body is attacked by the little living animals known as <u>germs</u>.

Germs live everywhere around us - in the air, in the ground, in water. They get into our body through any opening:

- through the nose with the air that we breath,
- through the mouth with what we eat and drink,
- through the skin:
  - when we hurt ourselves
  - when a mosquito bites us
  - when a dog bites us ...

TO PROTECT PEOPLE AGAINST GERMS

TEACH THOSE WHO LIVE IN YOUR VILLAGE:

TO EAT WELL,

TO WASH FOOD BEFORE COOKING,

TO DRINK CLEAN WATER OR OTHER FLUIDS,

TO WASH PROPERLY,

TO PROTECT THEMSELVES AGAINST MOSQUITOS, FLIES, ...

IN CASES OF FEVER CARRY OUT THE FOLLOWING INSTRUCTIONS:

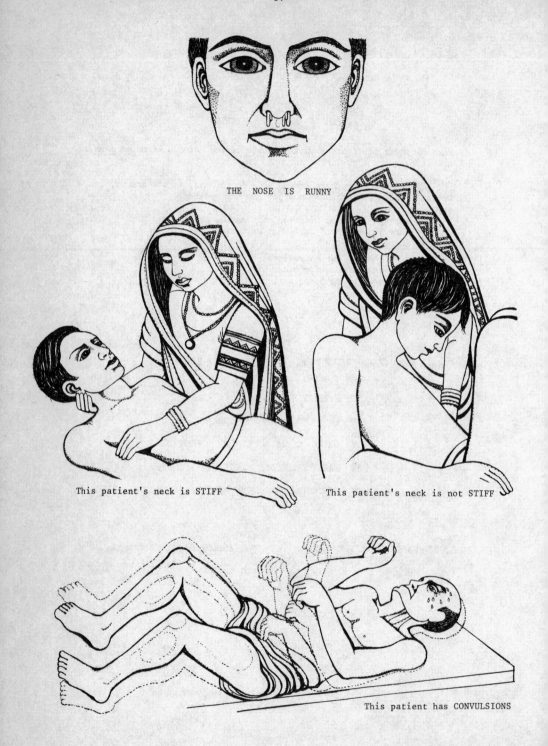

THE NOSE IS RUNNY

This patient's neck is STIFF

This patient's neck is not STIFF

This patient has CONVULSIONS

FEVER

Ask:

<u>How long</u> has the patient had a fever?

1.   <u>IF HE HAS HAD A FEVER FOR LESS THAN A WEEK</u>

Ask if:

      1.1 It started with a <u>runny nose</u>. Take the temperature,
      see page 252. See "The patient has been coughing or
      spitting for several days", page 29.

      1.2 If it did <u>not start with a runny nose</u>, either:

      1.2.1 The patient is <u>feverish and nothing else</u>.
      Always give <u>chloroquine</u> (see page 249).
      If the patient is under 5 years old, give <u>aspirin</u>
      (see page 249).

      or:

      1.2.2 The patient is <u>feverish with other signs</u>

      a) his neck is stiff (see drawing)
         or he does not move and does not answer when spoken to
         or he has convulsions (he does not answer and sometimes makes
            violent movements with the whole of his body or part of
            his body: face, arms, legs)
         or he is constantly vomiting.

         Give him an injection of <u>penicillin</u> (see page 251), and
         send him immediately to the hospital or health centre.

      b) if he has diarrhoea, spots on the skin, belly pains,
         pain in the joints ...

         See the corresponding problems.

2.   <u>IF HE HAS HAD A FEVER FOR MORE THAN A WEEK</u>

Send the patient to the hospital or the health centre.

DIARRHOEA

TO HAVE DIARRHOEA IS TO PASS AT LEAST THREE LIQUID STOOLS
PER DAY.

WHEN SOMEONE HAS DIARRHOEA, HE RAPIDLY LOSES WATER, SALT
AND STRENGTH.

TO TREAT DIARRHOEA IS TO GIVE THE PATIENT WATER, SALT AND
SUGAR AND TO TELL HIM TO EAT AS USUAL IN ORDER NOT TO LOSE
STRENGTH.

DIARRHOEA

LEARNING OBJECTIVES

At the end of his training, the PHW should be able to:

1. Identify four ways in which one may get diarrhoea

2. Demonstrate to the mother and community how to prevent
    diarrhoea

3. Decide whether a patient has diarrhoea or not

4. Recognize five major signs usually found in a person
    with a diarrhoea that indicate he should be sent
    to the hospital or health centre

5. Send to hospital or to a health centre any person
    with diarrhoea:
    - with dehydration, and
    - which does not respond to treatment in
      three days

6. Give oral fluid and diet treatment to both children
    and adults with diarrhoea

7. Show a mother whose child has diarrhoea how she should
    prepare and give oral fluid, and take care of her
    child

8. Show an adult patient and his attendants how to prepare
    and use oral fluid

DIARRHOEA

YOU GET DIARRHOEA FROM GERMS THAT ENTER YOUR BODY

- because you <u>drink water</u> which is <u>not clean</u> (from a pond, a river, a spring or a well which is not protected, water which has been kept in a dirty container),

- because you eat <u>dirty food</u> (badly washed, left outside or in a warm place for too long, not protected against flies and animals),

- because you eat certain foods which have <u>not</u> been <u>cooked long enough</u>,

- because you eat with <u>dirty hands</u> (after working or after defecating).

TO AVOID DIARRHOEA IN YOUR COMMUNITY TELL AND SHOW THE INHABITANTS HOW TO :

<u>*PREPARE AND CLEAN FOODS*</u>

<u>*GET CLEAN WATER*</u>

<u>*WASH HANDS BEFORE EATING AND AFTER DEFECATING*</u>

IF THERE IS A CASE OF DIARRHOEA TELL THE PATIENT AND HIS FAMILY ONCE AGAIN THAT THEY MUST CARRY OUT THE ABOVE INSTRUCTIONS.

THEN YOU SHOULD CARRY OUT THE INSTRUCTIONS ON THE FOLLOWING PAGES.

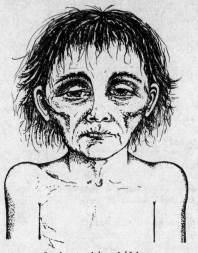 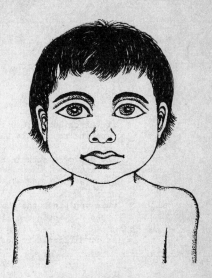

Look at this child:
his eyes are sunk in
  his head, his cheeks
  are hollow and his
  mouth is dry.

Look at this other child.
Is he different?

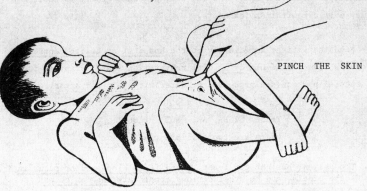

PINCH THE SKIN

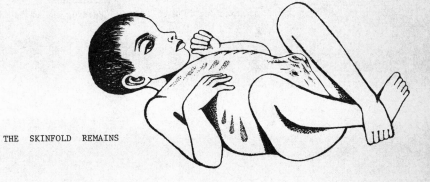

THE SKINFOLD REMAINS

DIARRHOEA

Examine the patient who has diarrhoea.

FIND OUT IF HE IS DEHYDRATED:

- if the child is less than eighteen months old, is the soft spot
  on the top of his head sunk in?

- are his eyes sunk in his head?

- are his mouth and his tongue dry?

- when you pinch the skin, does the skinfold remain for a few
  seconds instead of falling back again at once?

- is it difficult to feel the pulse on the wrist?

IF THESE SIGNS ARE PRESENT

BE CAREFUL: The situation is serious because the diarrhoea makes the
patient lose water and salt: he may die, and where there is cholera
he may even die within a few hours.

Send the patient immediately to the hospital or health centre.
Before he leaves make him drink oral rehydration fluid, prepared from
the special packet (see page 250) or water with salt and sugar.

IF THESE SIGNS ARE NOT PRESENT,
there are two possibilities:

1. The patient has not got fever, there is no blood and no mucus in
    the stools, and no other serious complaints such as cough

    1.1 The patient should continue to eat as usual
        If the patient is a child, see "Feeding the child" (page 84)

WHEN HE HAS DIARRHOEA CONTINUE TO

GIVE HIM SOMETHING TO DRINK

like this   or   like this

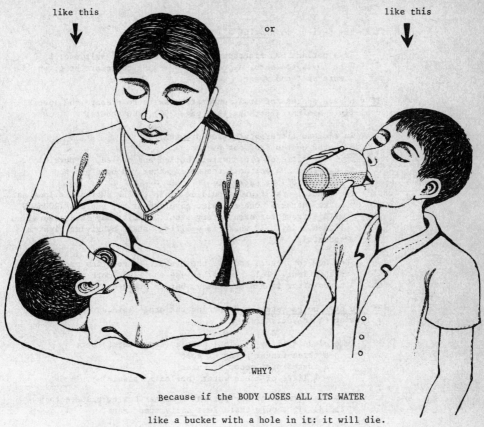

WHY?

Because if the BODY LOSES ALL ITS WATER

like a bucket with a hole in it: it will die.

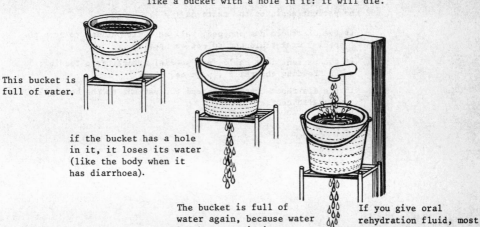

This bucket is
full of water.

if the bucket has a hole
in it, it loses its water
(like the body when it
has diarrhoea).

The bucket is full of
water again, because water
has been put in it.

If you give oral
rehydration fluid, most
diarrhoeas will soon
stop naturally.

DIARRHOEA

1.2 The patient must <u>drink a lot of liquid</u>

If a patient has diarrhoea, he loses water and salt and, if
he loses too much, he may die. He must therefore be given
more salt and water.

<u>If you have packets</u> of oral rehydration salts to prepare the special
oral fluid against diarrhoea (see page 250), you should:

In a clean litre bottle (see drawing) put:
    the contents of one packet,
    one litre of clean water (boiled and cooled, if possible).
Be careful: Do not boil the water after you have put the
    contents of the packet in it.
The special oral fluid should be given to the patient as long as
    he is thirsty. One can also give one or two cupfuls (200-400
    millilitres) for each watery stool. Adults may need several
    litres a day. If there is vomiting, start by giving sips or
    spoonfuls.

Show how to prepare and use the fluid. Leave a few packets with
    the patient. Tell him not to use the fluid more than 18 to 24
    hours after it has been made, but to prepare a fresh lot.

<u>If you have no packets</u> for preparing the oral fluid, prepare the
following fluid yourself:

In a clean ½ litre (1 pint) bottle (see drawing) put:
    a three-finger pinch of salt
    a four-finger scoop of sugar
    a ½ litre of clean water (boiled if possible).

Show the patient or the patient's mother how to prepare this
    fluid. It should taste <u>less salty</u> than tears.

<u>SEE</u> the patient again on the third day:

If the diarrhoea has stopped, tell an adult patient to stop the
    special oral fluid and to eat as usual.

If the patient is a child, pay special attention to feeding;
    see "Feeding the child", page 84.

If the diarrhoea continues, send the patient to the hospital
    or health centre.

TO PREPARE ORAL FLUID

FIRST OF ALL,
BOIL SOME WATER

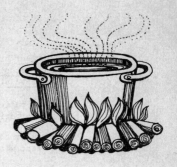

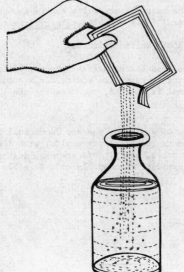

THEN, DO THIS

IF YOU HAVE NO PACKETS,
DO THIS

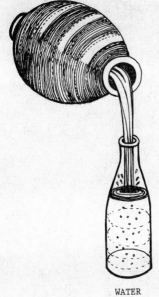

WATER   +   SALT   +   SUGAR

2. The patient has a high temperature (over 39°C), or blood and mucus
   in the stools, or other serious complaints like cough or more
   than five stools a day

   Send the patient to the hospital or health centre, but in the meantime
   make him drink a lot of oral fluid.

   If transfer to the hospital or health centre is not possible, continue
   to treat with oral fluid and give tetracycline (see page 251).

   SEE the patient AGAIN on the third day:

   - If the diarrhoea is better or has stopped, advise the patient
     to stop taking tetracycline and to eat as usual.
     If the patient is a child, see "Feeding the child", page 84.

   BE CAREFUL: If, at any time, you see an unusual increase in the
   number of patients (particularly adults) with diarrhoea, closely
   following each other, or if there are many deaths from diarrhoea
   - think of epidemics: see "Epidemics", page 37.

RESPIRATORY

DISEASES

A PATIENT WITH RESPIRATORY DISEASE COUGHS, AND WHEN HE COUGHS HE SPREADS LITTLE DROPS OF SPUTUM INTO THE AIR. THE PEOPLE WHO LIVE VERY CLOSE TO THE PATIENT BREATHE IN THIS AIR WHICH IS NOT CLEAN. THAT IS HOW CERTAIN CHEST DISEASES ARE SPREAD TO OTHER PEOPLE.

A PATIENT WHO HAS BEEN COUGHING OR SPITTING FOR YEARS MAY PASS ON SERIOUS DISEASES TO OTHER PEOPLE.

LEARNING OBJECTIVES

At the end of his training, the PHW should be able to:

1. Examine and find out from a patient if he has a
    cough

2. List two signs of mild (less than 38°C) respiratory
    infection

3. Treat a patient who has had a cough for some days
    with or without a temperature

4. List four signs of more serious respiratory infection
    (more than 38°C)

5. Treat patient with a temperature of more than 38°C
    with penicillin or sulfadiazine

6. Treat a child who coughs occasionally but turns blue
    and vomits

7. Decide when to send a patient to hospital or a health centre:

    7.1 any person who has had a cough for some days and
         is feverish but has not got better with treatment
    7.2 any child less than six months old with an occasional
         cough who becomes blue and vomits
    7.3 any patient who has had a cough for several weeks
         or several months,
              who spits blood,
              who has difficulty in breathing at night or
                 when walking,
              who has pains in the chest,
              who coughs up foul-smelling sputum

8. Tell the people three ways to prevent respiratory infection

YOU CATCH MOST RESPIRATORY DISEASES

- *because you live with people who are coughing and spitting; they are more serious for young people and people who are badly fed,* **because they are weaker and may die of them,**

- *because you are not warmly dressed during the day or not properly covered at night when it is cold.*

IN ORDER TO AVOID RESPIRATORY DISEASES IN YOUR VILLAGE, TELL AND REMIND THE PEOPLE THAT:

- *they should dress warmly when it is cold*
- *they and especially their children should eat well*
- *they should not cough on other people or children; they should not spit on the floor, especially in the house or in the hut. They should spit into a handkerchief, into a box or anything else which can be washed or burnt.*

When you are treating a PATIENT WITH A RESPIRATORY DISEASE,

TELL HIM AND REMIND HIM THAT:

HE AND HIS CHILDREN SHOULD EAT WELL

HE SHOULD NOT COUGH ON OTHER PEOPLE OR SPIT ON THE FLOOR

HE SHOULD TAKE GOOD CARE OF HIMSELF, ESPECIALLY WHEN THE PATIENT HAS BEEN COUGHING FOR A LONG TIME,

and carry out the following INSTRUCTIONS:

BE   CAREFUL:

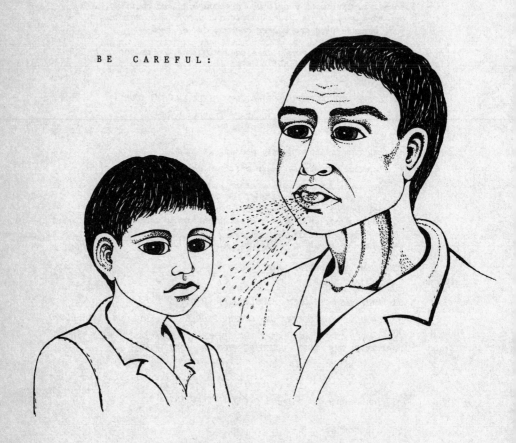

People, and especially CHILDREN, should not be allowed
too near PEOPLE who are coughing.

RESPIRATORY DISEASES

Examine the patient with respiratory disease, and always begin by asking him: "How long have you been coughing and spitting?"

1. IF THE PATIENT HAS BEEN COUGHING AND SPITTING FOR A FEW DAYS

    Take his temperature (see technique, page 252)

    1.1 The patient's temperature is less than 38°C

        - either he has a runny nose (with a discharge like water or
            a thicker discharge like milk)
        - or he has a sore throat every time he swallows anything.

        Give him aspirin for three days (see page 249)
        and tell him not to cough on other people, especially children,
        or spit on the floor.

        SEE the patient AGAIN on the fourth day:

        - everything is all right, the patient is cured. Tell him to
            come back if he becomes feverish; or
        - there is no improvement, and the patient is feverish:
            see 1.2.

    1.2 The patient's temperature is over 38°C

        - either the patient has difficulty in breathing, and breathes
            rapidly,
        - or his throat is very sore whenever he swallows anything,
        - or he has discharge from one ear,
        - or he has red spots all over his body and a runny nose and
            eyes

        Give him penicillin, or if you have none, sulfadiazine
        tablets (see page 251)*

        SEE the patient AGAIN on the third day:

        - everything is all right; the patient is cured; or
        - there is no improvement; send the patient to the hospital
            or the health centre.

    ---

    * If you have neither penicillin nor sulfadiazine, send the patient to
      the hospital or the health centre

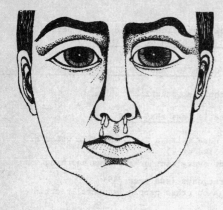

He has a runny nose

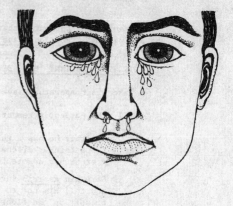

His nose and eyes are runny

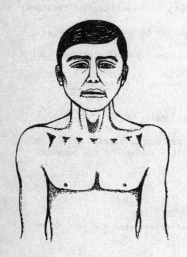

He has difficulty
in breathing

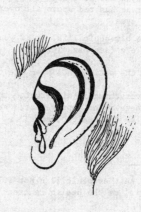

He has a discharge
from one ear

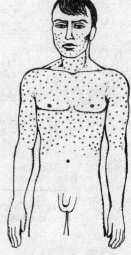

His body is covered in
little red spots

RESPIRATORY DISEASES

    1.3 If the patient is a child who had a runny nose to start with, but who, after a few days, coughs a lot at times, becomes all blue and vomits phlegm (sputum) or food.

       1.3.1 If the child is <u>less than 6 months old</u>
Send him to the hospital or the health centre.

       1.3.2 If the child is <u>over 6 months old</u>
Give him aspirin (see page 249)
But tell the mother that she should bring the child back to you if he becomes feverish
In that case, treat the child as in 1.2.

2.   <u>IF THE PATIENT HAS BEEN COUGHING AND SPITTING FOR WEEKS OR MONTHS</u>

Always send this patient to the hospital or health centre, because his illness could be serious, and ask him to come back and see you after he has been to the hospital or health centre. If he has been prescribed a treatment, make sure that he takes it regularly.

3.   <u>IF THE PATIENT IS SPITTING BLOOD, HAS DIFFICULTY IN BREATHING AT NIGHT OR WHEN WALKING, HAS A PAIN IN HIS CHEST OR COUGHS UP PHLEGM WHICH SMELLS BAD</u>

Whenever a patient shows any of these signs send him to the hospital or the health centre.

People who live with a patient who coughs and spits may catch his illness. They should also be examined and told to come and see you as soon as they start coughing or spitting.

———

VENEREAL

DISEASES

(or, sexually-transmitted diseases)

THESE ARE THE DISEASES WHICH A MAN AND A WOMAN MAY PASS ON TO EACH OTHER DURING SEXUAL INTERCOURSE WHEN ONE OF THEM IS INFECTED.

IN MANY PLACES THEY AFFECT A LARGE NUMBER OF YOUNG PEOPLE.

THEY HAVE SERIOUS CONSEQUENCES IF NOT TREATED IMMEDIATELY:

- *infection of the internal and external genitals*
- *sterility in the man and the woman*
- *miscarriage*
- *a baby may be born with a venereal disease if the mother has a venereal disease which has not been treated.*

VENEREAL DISEASES CAN BE EASILY TREATED AND CURED.

YOU SHOULD ALWAYS TREAT THE MAN AND THE WOMAN AT THE SAME TIME, IF POSSIBLE.

VENEREAL DISEASES

LEARNING OBJECTIVES

At the end of his training, the PHW should be able to:

1. Recognize three major signs of venereal disease

2. Treat a man who has a white/yellow discharge from the penis

3. Treat a woman who has a white/yellow discharge from the vagina

4. Tell when the patient is cured

5. Send to the hospital any patient who is not cured

6. Recognize the danger of a sore place on the genital organs

7. Treat a man or woman with sores on the genital organs

8. Explain to people how the disease is spread and how to avoid getting it

9. Give treatment to all sexual partners of a man or woman with a venereal disease.

VENEREAL DISEASES

A MAN OR A WOMAN COMES TO SEE YOU BECAUSE OF SOMETHING WRONG WITH THE GENITALS.

EITHER:

1. MOST COMMONLY, IT HURTS WHEN URINATING AND THERE IS A WHITE/YELLOW DISCHARGE THROUGH THE GENITALS (drawings 1 and 2)

   You should give the patient an injection of penicillin of 4 million units (four times 1 million units in the same syringe)

   If you have no penicillin, give the patient tetracycline tablets, 8 tablets a day for four days

   To all sexual partners in the past two weeks, give the same treatment.

   If the white/yellow discharge goes away five days after treatment, the patient is cured.

   Otherwise, send the patient to the hospital or health centre.

OR:

2. LESS COMMONLY, HE OR SHE HAS A SMALL SORE (ULCER) ON THE GENITALS (drawings 3 and 4)

   Later, the disease will continue even if the sore goes away without any treatment. For this reason, if you see the sore, you should treat it immediately and give the patient an injection of penicillin, 1 million units every day for ten days.

   To all sexual partners in the past month, give the same treatment.

   If you have no penicillin, or

   If the ulceration does not go away, send the patient to the hospital or the health centre.

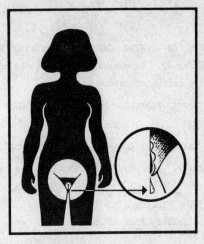

- 1 -

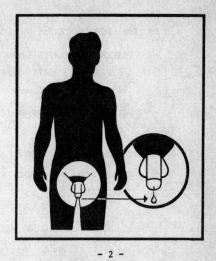

- 2 -

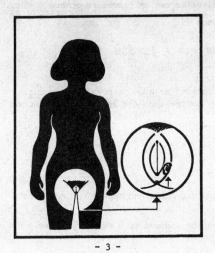

- 3 -

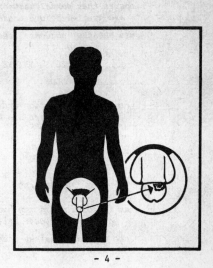

- 4 -

(Drawings by the Family Planning Association)

VENEREAL DISEASES

DO NOT FORGET THAT:

- VENEREAL DISEASES ARE PASSED ON DURING SEXUAL INTERCOURSE WITH
  PEOPLE WHO HAVE THESE DISEASES, *because they often do not know*
  they have the disease or they pay no attention to it

- SEXUAL INTERCOURSE WITH SEVERAL PARTNERS INCREASES THE RISK
  OF CATCHING THESE DISEASES

- IF THE GENITALS ARE NOT CLEAN, IT ALSO INCREASES THIS RISK.

- **THESE DISEASES CAUSE STERILITY, ABORTION AND INFECTION OF BABIES**
  AT BIRTH.

    TELL THE PEOPLE IN YOUR VILLAGE/DISTRICT
    THAT TO AVOID THESE DISEASES THEY SHOULD:

- *avoid sexual intercourse with people who have too many partners*
- *keep very clean by always washing their genitals with soap and*
  water after sexual intercourse
- *always urinate after sexual intercourse*
- **ensure that sexual partners of patients with venereal diseases**
  are treated before these diseases can be passed to others
- **use sheaths (condoms) (see page 75)**

    IF SOMEONE THINKS HE HAS A VENEREAL DISEASE,
    HE SHOULD:

- *come for examination and treatment as soon as possible, because*
  venereal diseases are easy to treat at the beginning, but more
  difficult later

    YOU SHOULD ALSO KNOW THAT:

- *an infected woman may have no discharge and may or may not have*
  pains in the lower belly
- *she may nevertheless pass on the disease to a sexual partner.*

EPIDEMICS

WHEN SEVERAL PEOPLE CATCH THE SAME DISEASE ABOUT THE SAME
TIME, IT IS CALLED AN EPIDEMIC.

IF THERE IS AN EPIDEMIC, YOU MUST NOT ONLY TREAT THE
PEOPLE WHO ARE ILL BUT ALSO PROTECT THE PEOPLE WHO ARE
HEALTHY SO THAT THEY DO NOT BECOME ILL.

LEARNING OBJECTIVES

At the end of his training, the PHW should be able to:

1. List four signs of illness which could cause an
    epidemic

2. List the precautions he would advise the community
    or person to take to prevent the spread of:

    2.1 diarrhoea
    2.2 respiratory diseases
    2.3 coughing and vomiting in children
    2.4 fever - with running nose and eyes and red spots
         on the skin, particularly in children

3. Advise patients and the community how to prevent the
    spread of skin disease with small blisters on the
    skin

4. Decide when to notify the supervisor about dangerous
    diseases or many people having the same disease

If there is an

EPIDEMIC

There are: 1. *People with diarrhoea (more than 3 liquid stools per day), or*

2. *People with a cough, or*

3. *People who are feverish and have spots on their skin, or*

4. *People who are feverish and do not have anything else. (see page 11)*

1. PEOPLE WITH DIARRHOEA

Children as well as adults.
It is almost always in hot weather that these cases occur.
To treat them, see "Diarrhoea",
But be careful! this disease is catching and may be dangerous.
Therefore, tell the people of your village:

1. To wash their hands before eating and after defecating

2. To drink only water that has been boiled

3. To eat only food that has been cooked

4. To use latrines if possible

5. To ask the village chief to help them build wells which will provide them with good water.

2. PEOPLE WITH A COUGH

2.1 Children and adults with runny noses and a cough

It is almost always in cold weather that these cases occur.
BE CAREFUL: this disease is catching and may be dangerous, especially for small children and old people.

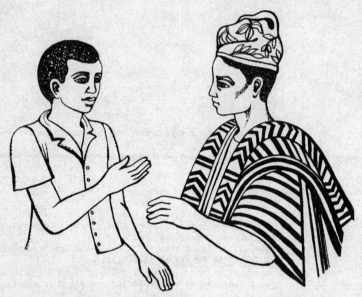

When there is an epidemic, you need the help of
other people: Talk to the village chief or to
the heads of families.   Inform the supervisor.

EPIDEMICS

To treat them, see "Respiratory diseases", page 25,
and tell the people living in your village:

1. To stay at home when they have a cough and a runny nose

2. Not to stay out in the cold and to wear enough clothes
   to keep them warm

3. To take good care of the children and old people, and to come
   to see you immediately if, after a few days, someone has a
   high temperature, difficulty in breathing or discharge from
   an ear.

2.2 Children have a bad cough, become blue in the face and vomit

To treat them, see "Respiratory diseases"
BUT BE CAREFUL: this disease is catching and may be dangerous,
especially for small children.
Therefore, tell the people of your village that:

1. If they have small children, they should not let them play
   with children who are ill

2. If they have children who are ill, they should keep them
   at home while they have a bad cough and are vomiting, and
   they should bring them to you immediately if they become
   feverish or have difficulty in breathing

and report the new cases to your supervisor every week.

3. PEOPLE WHO ARE FEVERISH AND HAVE SPOTS ON THEIR SKIN

3.1 They are children

3.1.1 Either they have a cough and a runny nose and eyes
To treat them, see "Respiratory diseases"
BUT BE CAREFUL: this disease is catching and may be dangerous
Therefore, tell the people of your village that:

1. If they have children, they should not let them play with
   children who are ill

2. If they have children who are ill, they should keep them at
   home while they have a fever and spots on their skin, and
   bring them to you immediately if they have difficulty in
   breathing.

and report the new cases to your supervisor every week.

3.1.2 Or they have something on the skin, but they do not have
       a cough or runny eyes
To treat them, see "Skin diseases" page 155.
Do not do anything unless your supervisor tells you.

3.2 They are adults

3.2.1 They have small watery blisters on the skin
BE CAREFUL: this disease may be dangerous.
Therefore, tell the people of your village that:

> if someone in their house is ill, they should keep him
> in bed and tell their neighbours and friends not to
> come to their house,

and report every new case to your supervisor.

3.2.2 It is something else
To treat them, see "Skin diseases"
and report the new cases to your supervisor every week.

PREGNANCY

PREGNANCY IS WHEN A WOMAN IS EXPECTING A BABY: SHE IS PREGNANT.

NORMALLY, A WOMAN WHO IS BETWEEN 15 AND 45 YEARS OLD LOSES BLOOD THROUGH THE VAGINA EVERY MONTH. THIS IS CALLED A PERIOD. WHEN SHE HAS NOT HAD A PERIOD FOR MORE THAN SIX WEEKS, SHE IS PROBABLY PREGNANT AND HER CHILD WILL BE BORN ABOUT NINE MONTHS AFTER THE DATE OF HER LAST PERIOD.

THE BABY DEVELOPS INSIDE THE MOTHER'S BELLY IN A POCKET KNOWN AS THE WOMB; AS THE CHILD GROWS, THE WOMB BECOMES BIGGER. YOU CAN FEEL IT WHEN YOU PUT YOUR HAND ON THE BELLY OF A WOMAN WHO IS MORE THAN THREE MONTHS PREGNANT.

PREGNANCY

LEARNING OBJECTIVES

At the end of his training, the PHW should be able to:

1. List two positive signs of pregnancy

2. Say after examination whether a woman is less than
    five months pregnant, or six months pregnant and
    over, or at term

3. Advise a pregnant woman on hygiene and nutrition

4. Treat a pregnant woman who complains of being tired
    with or without fever

5. Treat bleeding as prescribed

6. List three situations when a woman who is bleeding
    must be sent to the hospital or health centre

7. Decide by feeling the woman's belly whether it is
    hard or not

8. Describe four conditions in pregnancy when you must
    send the woman to the hospital or health centre

9. Send to the hospital or health centre any pregnant
    woman who:

    -   is suffering from vomiting
            directly if the vomiting occurs in the last
            four months of pregnancy
            after treatment has failed if vomiting occurs
            in the first five months
    -   is losing blood from below (the vagina)
    -   continues to feel tired after one month's treatment
    -   has a discharge which stains her underclothes and
            does not respond to treatment
    -   during the last four months of pregnancy has
            swollen legs, or a hard and tender belly

P R E G N A N C Y

Pregnancy is not a disease, but the diseases which occur during pregnancy may be dangerous because, if they affect the mother, they may also affect the child she is expecting.

PREGNANCY SHOULD THEREFORE BE SUPERVISED REGULARLY because a pregnancy which is not supervised may sometimes kill either the mother or the child or both of them.

YOU SHOULD TELL THE PEOPLE OF YOUR VILLAGE OR DISTRICT THAT ANY WOMAN UNDER ABOUT 45 YEARS OF AGE WHO HAS NOT HAD A PERIOD FOR OVER SIX WEEKS SHOULD COME AND SEE YOU TO FIND OUT IF SHE IS PREGNANT

AND IF SHE IS PREGNANT, TELL HER WHAT TO DO TO PROTECT HER HEALTH AND THE HEALTH OF THE CHILD SHE IS EXPECTING

EVERY TIME A PREGNANT WOMAN COMES TO SEE YOU, CARRY OUT THE FOLLOWING PROCEDURE:

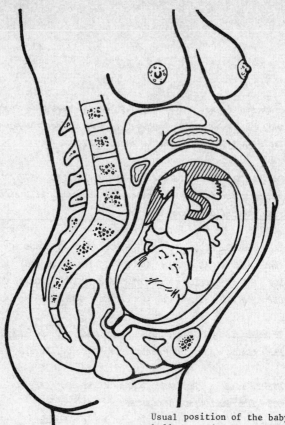

Usual position of the baby in its mother's
belly towards the end of pregnancy

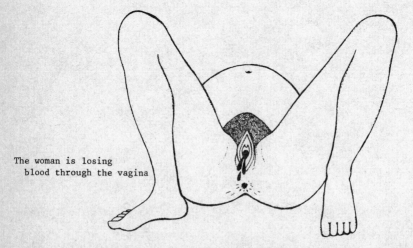

The woman is losing
blood through the vagina

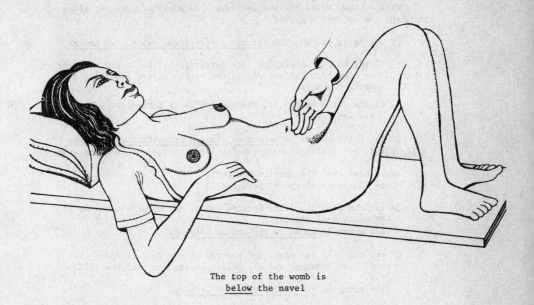

The top of the womb is
<u>below</u> the navel

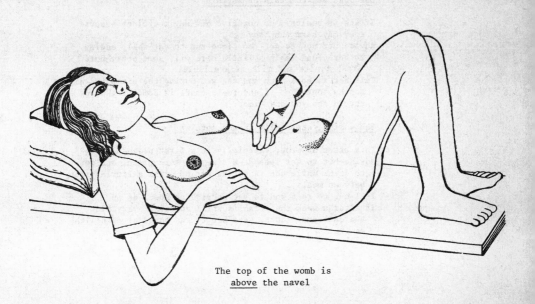

The top of the womb is
<u>above</u> the navel

When a woman tells you she no longer has a period, ask her <u>since</u> <u>when</u> she has not had a period.

If she tells you she has <u>not had a period for one to two months,</u>

- if she has no complaints, see paragraph 1.1 below and tell her to come back and see you in two months unless something goes wrong meanwhile

- if she has a complaint, see the following paragraphs 1.2, 1.3, 1.4 and 1.5

If she tells you it is <u>more than three months since she had her</u> <u>last period</u>, put your hand on her belly (see drawing) to feel the womb

You cannot feel the womb in her belly:
see "Diseases of women" paragraph 2.2

OR you can feel the womb, and the top of the womb is below or at the navel (see drawing):
This woman is <u>three to six months pregnant</u>

OR you can feel the womb, and the top of the womb is above the navel (see drawing) and she tells you she can feel the child move:
This woman is <u>six months pregnant or more</u>

1. <u>THE WOMAN IS THREE TO SIX MONTHS PREGNANT</u>

1.1 <u>She does not complain of anything</u>

If she is healthy, do not give her any medicines because they may harm the baby
Advise her not to get too tired and to eat well, adding to her usual meals a little more oil, some peas, nuts , fresh fruits and milk if available.
Tell her to come back and see you during the sixth and eighth months, but that if she feels there is something wrong she should see you any time.

1.2 <u>She vomits, especially in the morning</u>

This often happens, especially in a first pregnancy
Advise her to eat less at a time but more often, and not to drink while she is eating but to drink a little often between meals
Tell her to rest and to eat nourishing food, as in 1.1
If after a week the woman is still vomiting everything she eats and drinks, send her to the hospital or health centre.

1.3 She is losing blood through the vagina

1.3.1 She is losing no more blood than when she has her period, and her belly does not hurt

Tell her to stay in bed but to call you if she loses
   more blood
See her again the next day:
- she is losing less blood or no blood at all:
    tell her to rest as much as possible for a week
- she is no better, or she is losing blood again
    although she has not been losing any for several
    days:
    send her to the hospital or health centre and tell
    her to drink plenty of liquid on her way there.

1.3.2 She is losing more blood than when she has her period, and she has pains in the belly

Send her to the hospital or health centre and tell her
   to drink plenty of liquid on her way there

1.3.3 She has lost some blood but there were lumps in it like flesh

If she is no longer losing any blood, tell her that she
   probably had a miscarriage and that she must stay in
   bed and drink plenty of liquid.
See her again the next day. If she is losing more blood,
   give her 1 or 2 tablets of ergotamine (see page 250)
If the blood does not stop after one day, send her to
   the hospital or health centre
If she is no longer losing blood one day after she has
   taken the tablets, tell her to come back after one or
   two weeks to see if she is still pregnant (put your hand
   on her belly: where is the top of the womb?)
If she is no longer pregnant and she does not want another
   child for the time being, see "Family welfare"
If she is still pregnant, tell her to come back and see you
   during the sixth and eighth months and to eat well (see 1.1).

1.4 She feels tired and weak

Take her temperature

1.4.1 She is feverish:
See "Fever"

1.4.2 She is not feverish:
Advise her to eat well (see 1.1)
Give her iron sulfate tablets (see page 250)

1.5 She has belly pains

If she is losing blood, see 1.3
If she is not losing blood, see "Belly pains".

ADVISE
THE
PREGNANT WOMAN:

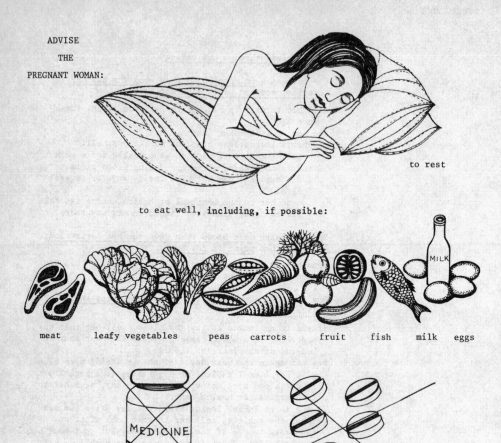

to rest

to eat well, including, if possible:

meat   leafy vegetables   peas   carrots   fruit   fish   milk   eggs

not to take any medicines without consulting the health personnel

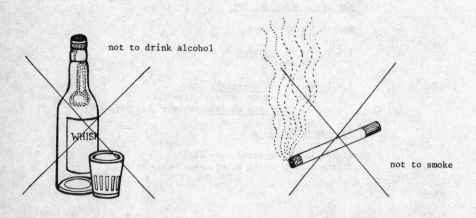

not to drink alcohol

not to smoke

ARE THE LEGS SWOLLEN?

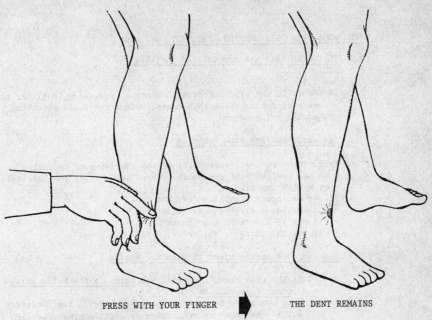

PRESS WITH YOUR FINGER ▶ THE DENT REMAINS

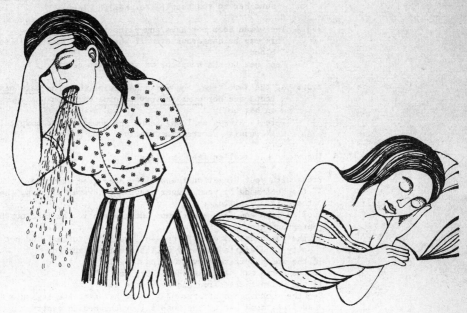

Vomiting is common
in early pregnancy

Advise her to rest

PREGNANCY

2. THE WOMAN IS SIX MONTHS PREGNANT OR MORE

2.1 The woman does not complain of anything

See 1.1
If she is in the sixth or seventh month of pregnancy, tell her to
come back during the eighth month, unless she feels something
abnormal before then.

2.2 The woman suffers from vomiting

This may be serious, especially if she complains of headaches
or has swollen feet and hands. Then, send her to the hospital
or health centre.
If she has not got swollen feet but
- if she has diarrhoea, see "Diarrhoea"
- if she is feverish, see "Fever"
- if she has pains in the belly, see "Belly pains".

2.3 The woman is losing blood through the vagina

2.3.1 At the same time, the woman has pains in the belly which
occur from to time
This woman may be ready to have her baby. See "Delivery".
But if the woman is only seven or eight months pregnant,
send her to the hospital or health centre.

2.3.2 The woman does not have any pains in the belly
This may be dangerous even if she is only losing a little
blood.
Send her to the hospital or the health centre

2.3.3 At the same time, the woman has pains, but the pain never
stops and her womb is very painful when you put your hand
on her belly
This is always serious: send the woman to the hospital or
the health centre immediately.

2.4 The woman has swollen feet and legs

Press with your finger on the swollen area (see drawing)
If the dent made by your finger stays for several minutes, then
there is a swelling
Swollen legs and feet are common among women in the last months of
pregnancy
If the woman has no other complaint, tell her to rest and not to eat
salty food and to put only a little salt on her food
If the woman suffers from vomiting, see 2.2
If the woman has pains in the belly, see 2.5
If the woman feels tired and weak, see 2.6
See the woman again after a week. If her feet and legs are still
swollen, send her to the hospital or the health centre
If the woman's face and hands are swollen, send her to the hospital
or the health centre.

2.5 The woman has belly pains

    2.5.1 If the pains come and go and then start again, and if her
            womb is hard but does not hurt, the woman is ready to have
            her baby. See "Delivery".

    2.5.2 If the pains continue without stopping and if her womb is
            painful when you put your hand on her belly, send the
            woman to the hospital or the health centre immediately.

    2.5.3 If the woman has a pain in the belly but her womb is not
            hard and does not hurt, see "Belly pains".

2.6 The woman feels tired and weak

See 1.4, but first ask her if she suffers from headaches or swollen
feet. If so, send her to the hospital or the health centre.

2.7 The woman is having or has just had convulsions

Make her lie down to ensure she will not fall. Make it possible
for her to breathe easily by trying to keep the mouth open and
clear from secretions.

This is always serious, so send the woman to the hospital or the
health centre as soon as possible.

———

DELIVERY

A NORMAL PREGNANCY LASTS ABOUT NINE MONTHS, AND THEN THE BABY COMES OUT OF THE MOTHER'S BELLY: THIS IS THE DELIVERY.

MOST DELIVERIES GO VERY WELL AND WITHOUT ANY DIFFICULTY. BUT ALL DELIVERIES SHOULD ALWAYS BE CAREFULLY SUPERVISED.

DELIVERY

LEARNING OBJECTIVES

At the end of his training, the PHW should be able to:

1. Decide whether labour is beginning or not

2. Send to the hospital or the health centre any woman in labour:
   - if the cord or the baby's hand or foot is the presenting part
   - if there is no presentation despite severe pains
   - if she is losing a lot of blood before or after the afterbirth (placenta) comes out

3. Take suitable measures of hygiene when labour begins

4. Recognize the presenting part

5. Break the bag of waters if necessary

6. Slow down the forward movement of the presenting part while supporting the woman's genitals

7. Deliver the baby

8. Tie and cut the cord

9. Clean out the baby's mouth after birth

10. Deliver the placenta

11. Say two things that should be done for a woman who has lost more than ½ litre of blood after the placenta comes out, before sending her to the hospital or health centre

12. List three signs of miscarriage (abortion).

D E L I V E R Y

Delivery is not a disease, but the accidents which may occur during delivery may be dangerous for the mother and the child.

DELIVERY SHOULD THEREFORE BE SUPERVISED or else the mother, or the child, or both, may die.

YOU SHOULD TELL THE PEOPLE WHO ATTEND DELIVERIES:

- TO KEEP THEIR <u>HANDS CLEAN</u>, TO USE CLEAN TOWELS AND CLEAN INSTRUMENTS (SCISSORS etc.)

- TO USE ONLY <u>CLEAN WATER</u>, BOILED IF POSSIBLE

- TO KEEP THE WOMAN AND THE CHILD CLEAN

- TO CALL YOU AS SOON AS SOMETHING UNUSUAL HAPPENS.

WHEN YOU ARE CALLED TO A DELIVERY, CARRY OUT THE FOLLOWING INSTRUCTIONS:

1. <u>How</u> can you <u>see</u> if the woman is about to have her baby?
2. What should you do <u>before</u> the baby comes out?
3. What should you do <u>while</u> the baby is coming out?
4. What should you do <u>after</u> the baby has come out?

WHAT TO DO BEFORE THE BABY COMES OUT

To begin with,
wash your hands and
forearms with soap
and water

then,
wash the woman's
genitals as well
... and your hands
once again

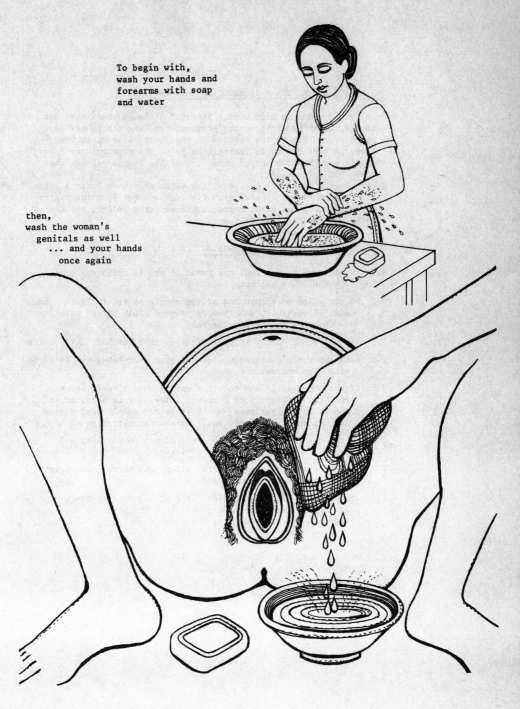

DELIVERY

1. HOW TO SEE IF THE WOMAN IS ABOUT TO HAVE HER BABY

Usually the woman is nine months pregnant although sometimes, but
rarely, seven or eight months pregnant, and she starts having
pains every five to ten minutes in the lower belly or in the
lower part of the back; during the pains the womb becomes hard.
A little pink fluid or blood comes out of the vagina as when the
woman has her period.
At the beginning of her delivery, the woman sometimes loses a large
quantity of water, "the waters" (it is the water from the bag in
which the baby has been living in his mother's belly), and the
pains will start soon afterwards.

2. WHAT TO DO BEFORE THE BABY COMES OUT

2.1 To begin with, reassure the woman if she is frightened and
    ask her to be patient

2.2 Do not allow more than one or two people to remain in the room
    and, if possible, ask them to prepare clean boiled water
    to wash the mother and the baby

2.3 Ask the woman to try to pass water so that her body will be free

2.4 Wash the woman's genitals and then wash your hands and forearms
    with soap and water

2.5 If the woman tells you that the waters have already broken,
    tell her to stay lying down until the baby is born, or in
    the squatting position, which is very commonly used and as
    safe as the lying position. Make a demonstration of both

2.6 If the waters have not yet broken, do not do anything and
    see 3. "While the baby is coming out"

2.7 Do not leave the woman once the pains have become more severe
    and occur every two minutes

2.8 If the pains become irregular, less strong or less frequent
    during the first 15 to 20 hours, send the woman to the
    hospital or health centre.

WHAT TO DO WHILE THE BABY IS COMING OUT

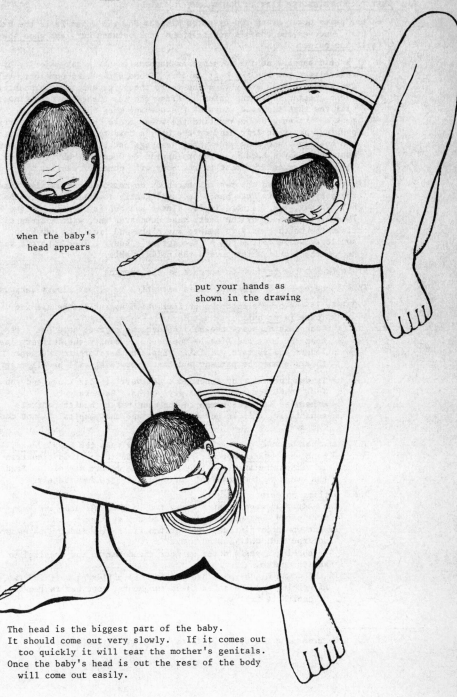

when the baby's
head appears

put your hands as
shown in the drawing

The head is the biggest part of the baby.
It should come out very slowly.   If it comes out
  too quickly it will tear the mother's genitals.
Once the baby's head is out the rest of the body
  will come out easily.

3.   WHAT TO DO WHILE THE BABY IS COMING OUT

When the pains occur every two or three minutes and the woman feels the need
to push, uncover the woman's genitals and look between her legs when she
feels the pains:

3.1 If a head appears at the opening, as happens in the great majority of
     deliveries: you can see hair on it.   To make the baby come out, tell
     the woman to push every time she feels the pains and to stop pushing when
     she no longer feels the pains.   After she has pushed several times, you
     will see that the head stays at the opening when the pains stop.   From
     that moment onwards, every time the woman feels the pains and starts
     pushing, put your left hand on the baby's head to stop it from coming out
     too quickly[1], and hook your right hand against the part of the woman
     where the baby's face is going to appear.   Once the baby's head is out,
     the shoulders and the rest of the body will come out easily.

     If the shoulders and the rest of the body do not come out easily, take
     the baby's head in both hands and pull gently downwards.   Once the
     baby is out, tie the cord in two places and cut it between the two knots.
     Then lift the baby by the feet, head downwards and, with a clean cloth,
     clean the mouth gently to remove any blood and liquid he may have
     swallowed while coming out of the mother's body.   Then wipe off very
     gently the liquid which covers the child's skin.

3.2 If it is not the head which appears at the opening

     This is rare, but BE CAREFUL: this situation is almost always serious

     3.2.1 It is the baby's buttocks or feet which appear at the opening.
           There is no hair.
           When this happens, the baby's buttocks or feet come out first,
           then the body and finally the head.   Usually the delivery lasts
           longer and is more painful.   Explain therefore to the woman
           that she must be patient and that everything will be all right.

           If you have already attended a delivery of this kind, and you
           feel confident, act in the way you have been taught.
           Otherwise send the woman to the hospital or health centre,
           especially if it is her first baby and the hospital is not too
           far away.

     3.2.2 Another unusual but serious situation is when the baby's cord,
           hand or shoulder appears first.   BE CAREFUL: this situation
           is serious because the baby and/or the mother may die.   Send
           the woman to the hospital or health centre immediately.

     3.2.3 Nothing appears
           The woman has severe pains every two to three minutes and even
           more often, but nothing appears at the opening.
           If the woman is giving birth for the first time and the pains are
           not too bad, wait for an hour.
           If nothing appears after an hour, send her to the hospital or
           health centre.
           If the woman has already had one or more children, wait for two hours.
           If nothing appears after these two hours, send her to the hospital
           or health centre.

---

[1] If the baby comes out too quickly, it may tear the mother's genitals.

WHAT TO DO AFTER THE BABY HAS COME OUT

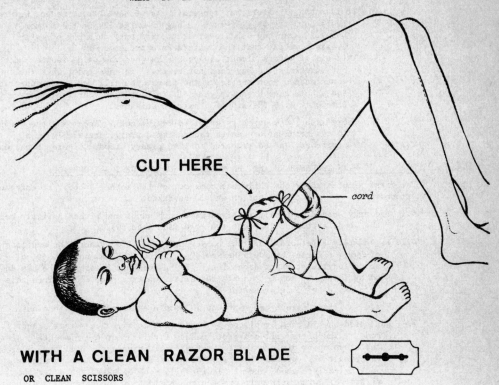

CUT HERE

cord

WITH A CLEAN RAZOR BLADE

OR CLEAN SCISSORS

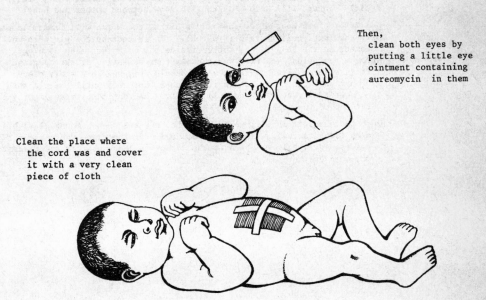

Then,
 clean both eyes by
 putting a little eye
 ointment containing
 aureomycin in them

Clean the place where
 the cord was and cover
 it with a very clean
 piece of cloth

3.2.4 It is a <u>bag of water</u> that appears. As we have already seen, before
he is born the baby lives in a bag of water inside the mother's
belly. When the baby is about to come out, this bag of water
breaks: we say that the "waters have broken".
This bag of waters almost always breaks when the pains become bad,
but sometimes the bag does not break. In this case, when the
woman pushes when she feels the pains, you will see a bag appearing.
You should then break it yourself, either with your finger or very
carefully with the tip of a pair of scissors.

3.2.5 There is a large <u>quantity of blood</u> coming out. Accompany the woman
to the hospital or health centre immediately, preferably on a
stretcher, and be prepared to give plenty of warm liquid on the way.

4. WHAT TO DO WITH THE NEWBORN AND THE MOTHER, ONCE THE BABY HAS COME OUT

The first minutes after the child has come out of the mother's body are extremely
important. Simple timely action should be taken:

4.1 The baby should be gently received with both hands and placed a little below
the level of the belly; cut the cord (see page 60).

4.2 Immediately afterwards, dry the baby gently to avoid evaporation and loss
of heat. Clean the mouth and nose. If the baby has not yet cried,
watch for the start of breathing. If he does not breathe, make him do
so by immediate mouth-to-mouth resuscitation (see page 92), since this
is a matter of life or death.

4.3 Place a little aureomycin ointment in both eyes to prevent infections.

4.4 The child should then be placed in close contact with the mother's nude
body. <u>The belly will contract</u>, making expulsion of the placenta easier
and stopping or diminishing the mother's bleeding after delivery, and
the breast will produce the first drops of milk. If the baby starts
sucking early, "good" breast feeding will soon be established and the
first, yellowish milk will protect the child from infections. This
early contact will help to establish love between mother and baby.

4.5 A quarter of an hour after the baby's birth, the woman will feel mild pains
in the lower belly; this is normal. It is because the <u>placenta</u> which
connected the baby to the mother inside the womb must also come out.
After a few pains, you will see the placenta appearing at the opening.
It is a large piece of flesh which should come out in a whole piece.
<u>Do not pull</u> the cord because it may tear, but wait until the placenta
comes out by itself. The only thing you can do is to press lightly on
the top of the womb.

4.6 Once the placenta is out, go back to the baby and wash him and clean his
eyes (see drawing). Then put a bandage over the place where the cord
was (see drawing). Return to the mother to check whether the placenta
was complete.

4.7 If the placenta has not come out an hour after baby's birth, or if the
mother is losing blood through the vagina, gently massage the top part
of the womb or, if you have any, give her an injection of <u>oxytocin</u>
in the buttock (see page 250).
If the placenta has not come out two hours after the baby's birth, or if
only part of it has come out, or if the mother is losing more blood,
send her to the hospital or health centre.

4.8 It is normal that the mother should lose about half a litre of blood
before and while the placenta comes out. But it is not normal that
she should lose more blood once the placenta has come out; if she does,
you should either gently massage the top of the womb or give her a
injection of <u>oxytocin</u>, as indicated in 4.7.
If the woman continues to lose blood, give her plenty of liquid to drink
and send her to the hospital or the health centre.

YOU SHOULD ALSO KNOW THAT:

- *WHEN A WOMAN WHO IS TWO TO SIX MONTHS PREGNANT LOSES
  BLOOD WHETHER IT IS PAINFUL OR NOT, WHICH CONTAINS
  LUMPS OF FLESH OR A SMALL DEAD BABY: THIS IS A
  MISCARRIAGE. SHE IS NO LONGER PREGNANT.*

- *WHEN A WOMAN GIVES BIRTH AFTER SEVEN OR EIGHT MONTHS,
  THE BABY WILL BE SMALLER AND WEAKER THAN A BABY BORN
  DURING THE NINTH MONTH OF PREGNANCY. IF HE IS NOT
  WELL LOOKED AFTER THIS BABY MAY DIE MORE EASILY
  BECAUSE HE IS NOT AS STRONG AS A FULL-TERM BABY.*

AFTER THE

DELIVERY

(or, postnatal care)

THE PERIOD AFTER THE DELIVERY IS THE PERIOD LASTING FORTY DAYS AFTER THE BIRTH OF THE BABY.

THE MOTHER'S BREASTS WILL PROVIDE MILK TO FEED THE BABY AND THE WOMB WILL BECOME SMALL AGAIN AS IT WAS BEFORE PREGNANCY.

FOR THE BABY, LIFE IS BEGINNING.

POSTNATAL CARE

LEARNING OBJECTIVES

At the end of his training, the PHW should be able to:

1. Determine the position of the top of the uterus

2. Advise and teach about cleanliness and good food

3. Treat a woman who has constipation

4. Recognize a raised temperature and give correct
    treatment

5. Treat pains in the lower belly, breasts, or legs

6. Recognize when treatment has not improved the condition

7. Recognize by feeling the belly when the uterus becomes
    normal

8. Recognize sudden and heavy bleeding. Give necessary
    treatment and SEND TO HOSPITAL

9. Send to the hospital or health centre any woman who has had
    a baby and whose fever or pains have not responded to
    treatment

A F T E R   T H E   D E L I V E R Y

During the month following the delivery you should tell the mother how to protect her health and that of her baby:

- *BY KEEPING HER BODY CLEAN*
- *BY KEEPING HER BABY CLEAN*
- *BY EATING WELL*
- *BY FEEDING HER BABY WELL*

This is when you should advise the woman and her husband to delay the next child, that is:

TO WAIT FOR A FEW YEARS BEFORE HAVING ANOTHER BABY

so that the mother will have enough time to get her strength back without tiring herself out with a new pregnancy while she is still feeding her baby, and so that the baby will be better fed and better looked after by his mother.

YOU SHOULD THEREFORE EXPLAIN TO THE WOMAN AND HER HUSBAND

WHAT TO DO TO AVOID HAVING CHILDREN FOR AS LONG AS THEY WISH

(See Problem 2.4 "Family welfare").

When you see a woman who has just had a baby,

CARRY OUT THE FOLLOWING INSTRUCTIONS:

POSTNATAL CARE

1. The mother has no complaints

or *2. The mother is feverish*

or *3. The mother has some other complaint.*

---

1. **THE   MOTHER   HAS   NO   COMPLAINTS**

1.1 She had her baby one or two days ago
Normally:
The womb is hard and the top of the womb is at the same level as the
   navel (see drawing).
Her breasts are beginning to produce milk.
The woman loses blood which is very red through her vagina, usually
   more than when she has her period.

Advise her:
1.   to feed her baby whenever he seems to want it, starting
     as soon as possible after birth
2.   to wash carefully every day with soap and water: her baby,
     her breasts and her genitals
3.   to eat well as during her pregnancy (see 1.1 page 48)
4.   to walk about a little, but not to tire herself
5.   if she feels mild pains in the belly, give her some aspirin
     for one or two days
6.   if she is constipated, advise her to eat fruit with her break-
     fast, to try to defecate in the morning after she has eaten,
     even if she does not need to, and to drink a big glass of
     water when she gets up in the morning and goes to bed at
     night.

1.2 She had her baby a week ago

The top part of the womb is between the navel and the hairs
   (see drawing)
The woman loses through her vagina a liquid which is at first brown
   and then a yellowish white
The baby sucks well
The cord became dry and fell off by itself

Advise her:
1.   to feed her baby well whenever he seems to want it,
     even during the night
2.   to wash her baby well, as well as her own breasts and genitals,
     with soap and water
3.   to go back to her ordinary work little by little, without
     tiring herself too much
4.   to go back to her usual diet again and adding, if possible, beans,
     cereals, eggs, meat, fish, vegetables and fresh fruit and
     milk if available
5.   not to have another baby for a few years. (See "Family
     welfare" page 73).

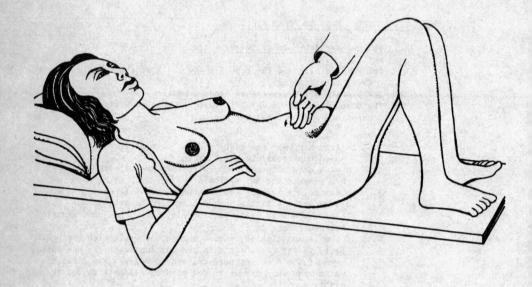

She had her baby a week ago

One or two days after the birth the womb reached to the navel; now, the top part of the womb is below the navel.

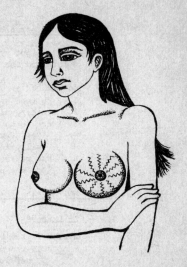

One breast hurts a lot

Tell the mother to squeeze the milk
from the breast with her hand and
to then give this milk to her baby

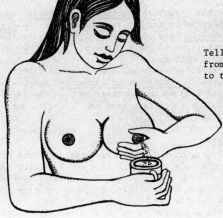

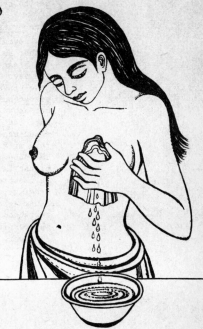

She should put hot compresses on the
breast that hurts: 3 or 4 thicknesses
of cloth dipped into hot water (but
not burning hot!)   She should do
this for 10 minutes and do it about
3 or 4 times a day

POSTNATAL CARE

1.3 <u>She had her baby about forty days ago</u>

When you put your hand on her belly you cannot feel the womb any
   more and the woman has no discharge from her vagina any more

Advise her:
1.   to feed her baby well and to wash him carefully
2.   to eat well, not to get too tired and to wash carefully
3.   not to have another baby for a few years
       See "Family welfare" page 73. Tell her that her period
       will start again in six to eight months time, but that
4.   she may become pregnant at any time if she or her husband
       do not use certain methods to avoid another pregnancy.

2.   <u>THE MOTHER IS FEVERISH</u>

2.1 <u>With pains</u>

   2.1.1   In the <u>belly</u>:
            If the woman has a vaginal <u>discharge which smells bad</u> and
            her womb hurts when you put your hand on her belly, give
            her some <u>aspirin</u> (see page 249) and at the same time, if
            you have some, one to two tablets of <u>ergotamine</u> (see page 250)
            See her again next day:
            If she is still feverish and her belly still hurts a little,
            give her some <u>penicillin</u> or <u>sulfadiazine</u>, and see her again
            every day as long as she is feverish. If she is still
            feverish on the fifth day, send her to the hospital or
            health centre.

   2.1.2   In one <u>breast</u>:
            It is normal that on the second or third day after birth the
            mother should be a little feverish and feel some pain in
            the breasts which are swollen. She is only feverish for
            one day: if her breasts hurt, give her a little <u>aspirin</u>
            If she stays feverish or becomes feverish again, and if <u>one
            breast</u> hurts a lot and is so painful that she cannot feed
            her baby: ask her to press her breast with her hand to
            make the milk come out. She must do this cleanly, with
            clean hands and using a clean glass. She should then give
            this milk to her baby. If she prefers, she can breast-feed
            the baby long enough and often enough to keep the painful
            breast fairly empty. Tell her also to put hot compresses
            on the breast which hurts, three to four times a day (see
            drawing), and give her some <u>aspirin</u>.
            See her again on the fourth day. If one of her breasts still
            hurts and contains a little lump which hurts, send her to
            the hospital or health centre.

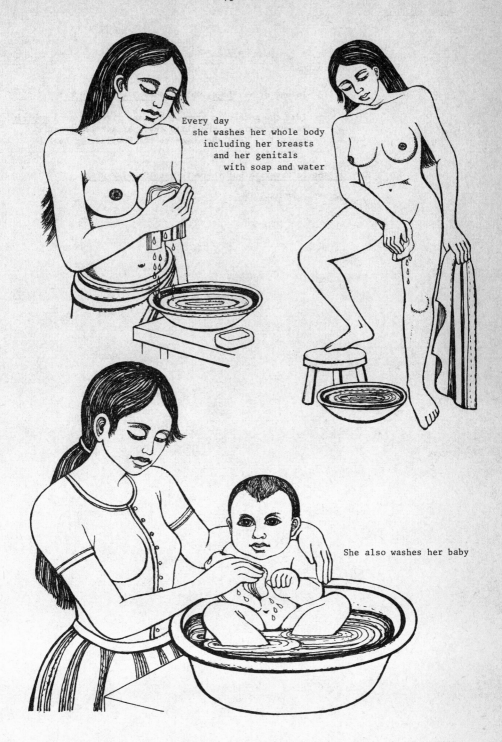

Every day
she washes her whole body
including her breasts
and her genitals
with soap and water

She also washes her baby

2.1.3 In one of her legs, which is swollen and hurts:

Tell the mother to stay in bed and give her some aspirin.
See her again on the third day. If her leg is still
swollen, send the woman to the hospital or health
centre.

2.2 If she is feverish but there is nothing else wrong

See "Fever" page 11.

FAMILY

WELFARE

FAMILY WELFARE IS EVERYTHING WHICH MAKES A FAMILY HAPPY. A FAMILY IS NOT HAPPY IF THE PARENTS AND THE CHILDREN ARE ILL, BADLY FED, TOO TIRED, TOO WEAK.

A WOMAN CAN HAVE A LOT OF CHILDREN, BUT SHE MAY WISH TO WAIT FOR A WHILE BEFORE HAVING ANOTHER ONE OR SHE MAY NOT WANT ANY MORE.

WHEN A WOMAN DOES NOT HAVE A CHILD EVERY YEAR, SHE WILL BE HEALTHIER AND SO WILL HER CHILDREN.

THERE ARE METHODS WHICH ALLOW A COUPLE EITHER TO HAVE A CHILD ONLY WHEN THEY WISH TO OR TO HAVE NO MORE CHILDREN.

FAMILY WELFARE

LEARNING OBJECTIVES

At the end of training, the PHW should be able to:

1. Talk with village people about why it is important for a woman to rest after having a baby

2. List three ways to avoid having a baby

3. Point to the contraceptives that a PHC may give to a woman or a man

4. Recognize when a woman is sick after taking contraceptive pills

5. Recognize when a woman, who is taking contraceptive pills or who has a coil, is sick and must go to the hospital because:
   - she has headaches and/or swollen legs
   - the coil has come out of the body

6. Talk with men about using a condom and how to make sure it is in good order

7. Refer to the health centre men and women who have problems because they do not want any more children

FAMILY WELFARE

The mother is a very important member of the family: she gives
birth to the children and she brings them up.   If her health is bad because
she eats badly or because she is too often pregnant, the health of her baby
will also be bad.

The father is the head of the family.   If he does not want his wife
to use a method of avoiding pregnancy, his wife **may** not want to either.

If you cannot inform and convince the father and sometimes even the
mother-in-law as well as the mother herself of the advantages of family
planning, you will very probably be wasting your time!

The village birth attendant is widely respected in the community
where she lives and works.   She probably delivers most of the babies.
It is important for you to be on good terms with her and to make
her understand what you are doing so that she can help you and give
the same advice as you do to the village people.

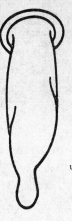

unrolled sheath
(or condom)

rolled-up sheath

A WOMAN AND HER HUSBAND MAY WISH TO WAIT FOR A WHILE BEFORE HAVING A BABY OR MAY WISH NOT TO HAVE ANY MORE.

When you see a woman again after a delivery or after a miscarriage, tell her and her husband, and also the other women living in the house, how it is possible to avoid becoming pregnant. But explain to them what to do, by showing them the drawings and the methods used.

1. **THE COUPLE WISH TO WAIT FOR A FEW YEARS BEFORE HAVING ANOTHER BABY**

    1.1 If they wish to use <u>sheaths</u>, explain to the husband how to use a sheath and give him ten. Tell him to come back in a few week's time before using the last sheath. If he is satisfied, give him more and tell him to come back for more before using all of those you have given him.
    If he is not satisfied, send the woman to the health centre so that she can learn how to take the pills or be fitted with a coil.

    1.2 If they do not want to use sheaths, send the woman to the health centre to get the pills or a coil.

    1.3 If the woman has been given <u>pills</u> at the health centre, see her again after a month and ask her how she is feeling.

    1.3.1 If she feels well, give her pills for three months and tell her to come back before she has used all of them.

    1.3.2 If she feels tired or if she loses a little blood through her vagina when she does not have her period, reassure her and tell her that these complaints will soon go away. Give her pills for two months and tell her to come back when she has finished them. If after these two months she still has the same complaints, send her to the health centre for consultation.

    1.3.3 If she complains of bad headaches, or if one of her legs is swollen and hurts, send her to the hospital or the health centre.

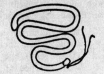

a <u>coil</u>
which is put in the womb

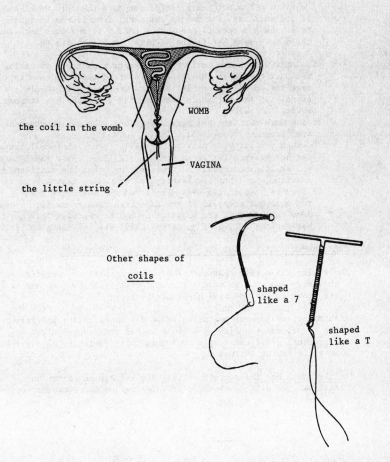

the coil in the womb

WOMB

VAGINA

the little string

Other shapes of
<u>coils</u>

shaped
like a 7

shaped
like a T

1.4 If the woman has been fitted with a <u>coil</u>, see her again after one month and ask her how she is feeling.

    1.4.1 If she has no complaints, see her again after three months and again after six months

    1.4.2 If the coil has come out of the vagina by itself, send her to the health centre to be fitted with a new one.

    1.4.3 If she complains of losing blood when she does not have her period or of having a discharge which is not blood, or of having had a very heavy period during the first month, reassure her and tell her that everything almost always stops after one or two months

        See her again after two months: if she is no better, send her to the hospital or health centre.

1.5 If the woman has not had a period for more than six weeks and she is not suckling, she may be pregnant, even if she is taking pills or if she has been fitted with a coil. If she does not want a child now, send her to the hospital or health centre.

1.6 If, later, the woman tells you she wants a baby but is taking pills, tell her to finish those she has started and then to stop. Her next period will probably be a few weeks late if she is not pregnant. See her again three months after she has stopped taking the pills.

If she does not have her period any more, she may be pregnant. See "Pregnancy" page 43.

If, when you put your hand on her belly, you cannot feel the womb, see her again after three months. If after these three months you still cannot feel the womb and the woman has still not had a period, send her to the hospital or health centre.

If she has been fitted with a coil and she now wants a baby, take the coil out yourself if you have been taught how to; if not, send the woman to the hospital or health centre. Tell her that her periods will come as before until she becomes pregnant.

2. <u>THE COUPLE NEVER WANT TO HAVE ANY MORE CHILDREN</u>

Explain to the couple that either of them can have an operation so that they can have no more children. If they wish, send one or the other to the hospital or health centre.

If the husband has the operation, give him some sheaths and instruct him to use one the first ten times he has intercourse after the operation. Tell the couple that there will no longer be any risk of their having children.

If the woman has the operation, tell her she can no longer have children but will continue to have her period as before her operation.

———

DISEASES

OF

WOMEN

WOMEN HAVE DISEASES WHICH MEN DO NOT HAVE; THEY ARE THE DISEASES WHICH AFFECT THOSE PARTS OF THEIR BODIES WHICH PRODUCE BABIES.

WOMEN LOSE SOME BLOOD FOR A FEW DAYS EVERY MONTH DURING THE YEARS WHEN THEY CAN HAVE BABIES. THIS LOSS OF BLOOD IS CALLED A PERIOD OR MENSTRUATION. WHEN A WOMAN'S PERIOD DOES NOT COME SHE IS PROBABLY EXPECTING A BABY. SHE IS THEN SAID TO BE PREGNANT, AND THIS CONDITION IS KNOWN AS PREGNANCY.

ANY WOMAN WHO LOSES BLOOD WHEN SHE IS NOT HAVING HER PERIOD, OR WHEN SHE NO LONGER HAS ONE, SHOULD ALWAYS BE SENT TO THE HOSPITAL OR THE HEALTH CENTRE.

DISEASES OF WOMEN

LEARNING OBJECTIVES

At the end of training, the PHW should be able to:

1. Advise any girl who complains she has not yet started
    her periods

2. Treat any girl who has painful periods

3. Tell if a woman is pregnant

4. Tell if a woman has reached an age when she can no
    longer have children

5. Advise a woman who is depressed, sleeps badly and
    complains that she hurts all over

6. Send to the hospital or health centre:

    - any girl who has not started her periods by the
      age of 16 years
    - any woman aged less than 40 years who no longer
      has her periods but who is not pregnant
    - any woman who is losing blood between her periods
      from below or who has discharges that stain her
      underclothes
    - any woman who has painful periods
    - any woman who remains depressed in spite of
      treatment

WOMEN MAY HAVE CERTAIN DISEASES IN THEIR GENITALS:

- *because they were not supervised or treated properly when they were expecting or when they had a baby (bad diet, bad hygiene, ...)*

- *because they have given birth to many babies, which injured their genitals*

and these diseases are often serious because women, who may not like to mention them, leave these diseases for too long before getting them treated.

TO PROTECT THE WOMEN IN YOUR VILLAGE OR IN YOUR DISTRICT AGAINST THESE DISEASES, ADVISE:

- *the women to get treated every time they are expecting a baby or when something goes wrong with their genitals*

- *the people who attend deliveries to keep their hands clean and to use clean utensils and instruments (to cut the cord, to wash the woman's genitals, ...)*

WHEN A WOMAN COMES TO SEE YOU BECAUSE OF A DISEASE IN HER GENITALS,

carry out the FOLLOWING INSTRUCTIONS:

DISEASES OF WOMEN

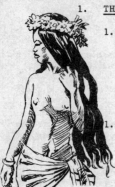

1. THE PATIENT IS A GIRL WHO HAS NOT YET STARTED HER PERIODS

1.1 She does not complain of anything

If the girl is not yet 16 years old, do nothing and tell the
family to bring her back when she is 16; advise them to
feed her well
If the girl is 16 years old or more, send her to the hospital
or health centre.

1.2 She has a complaint

For example, she has a cough, she is feverish, she feels tired,
she has pains in her belly. In this case, see the correspondi
PROBLEMS.

2. THE PATIENT IS A WOMAN WHO HAS NOT HAD HER PERIOD FOR AT
LEAST ONE MONTH

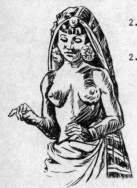

2.1 If she has not had her period for only one month:
Do nothing and tell her to see you after two months

2.2 If she has not had her period for three months or more:
Look for signs of pregnancy in the belly and see "Pregnancy"
If the woman is not pregnant, ask her if she sometimes feels
hot flushes which come up from her body towards her head,
as if she were feverish
If the woman tells you she sometimes feels hot flushes,
explain to her that it is because she has reached an age
when her body can no longer produce children. Advise her
to continue with her work but, if she is too fat, tell her
to eat less, especially less fatty or sugary food, such as
fried food, fatty meat, cakes.
If the woman tells you she does not feel these hot flushes,
send her to the hospital or health centre.

3. THE PATIENT IS A WOMAN WHO HAS PAINS IN HER BELLY EVERY
TIME SHE HAS HER PERIOD

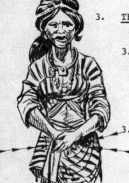

3.1 She is a girl or a woman who has not yet had any children:
Tell her to take aspirin during the first two days of her
period

If she is no better after a few months, send her to the hospit
or health centre

3.2 She is a woman who already has one or more children:
Send her to the hospital or health centre

DISEASES OF WOMEN

4. <u>THE PATIENT LOSES EITHER BLOOD OR SOMETHING ELSE</u>
   <u>THROUGH THE VAGINA</u>

The woman loses:

- blood when she does not have or no longer has her periods
- too much blood during her period
- something other than blood: such as water or pus

Send the patient to the hospital or the health centre, but if she is
losing a lot of blood, make her drink plenty of water.

5. <u>THE PATIENT IS A WOMAN WHO FEELS SAD AND TIRED</u>

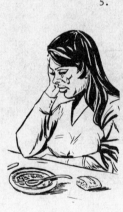

The woman is sad and cries a lot, she cannot sleep, and when she gets
up in the morning she already feels tired as if she had worked during
the night.
The patient will tell you that she can sometimes feel her heart beating
too hard in her chest; that her head, her arms, her legs hurt;
she has pains all over.

Talk to this woman who feels unhappy and try to find out why she is
sad

- It is because she does not want to have another baby, because
  she already has too many, because she has not enough money to
  feed them or to bring them up: see "Family welfare"
- OR, it is because she has problems in her life: in her work, with her
  husband, her children, her family, her neighbours:

Try to help her find a solution to her problem: talk to her husband
about it, for example. See "Mental disorders".

If, despite your advice, she is no better, send the patient to the
hospital or the health centre.

FEEDING

THE

CHILD

FOR A CHILD TO BE HEALTHY, HIS MOTHER SHOULD GIVE HIM HER MILK.

- NOTHING BUT MOTHER'S MILK DURING THE FIRST FOUR MONTHS

- THEN, FROM THE FIFTH MONTH TO A YEAR, HER MILK TOGETHER WITH OTHER FOODS.

WHEN THE CHILD IS ONE YEAR OLD, HE WILL EAT WHAT EVERYONE ELSE EATS.

MOTHER'S

MILK

IS

BEST

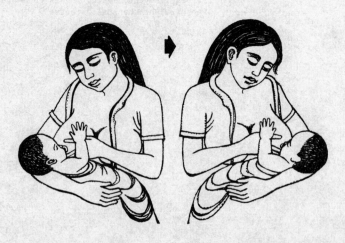

FEEDING THE CHILD

LEARNING OBJECTIVES

At the end of his training, the PHW should be able to:

1. List four reasons why breast-feeding is best for babies

2. Teach mothers breast-feeding techniques and sound practices

3. Say at which age a baby needs other foods as well as breast milk

4. List the food to give to a baby aged:

   4 months
   5 months
   1 year

5. Demonstrate how to prepare food for a baby aged five months and a baby aged one year

6. Weigh a child, write the weight on the Growth Chart and say if the child is on "the right road" or not

FEEDING THE CHILD

FOR A CHILD, MOTHER'S MILK IS BEST

- *because there is nothing better for making the baby grow in size and weight*

- *because it is always <u>clean</u> and needs <u>no preparing</u>*

- *because it does <u>not cost anything</u>*

- *because it protects the child against germs and diseases.*

TELL AND ALWAYS REMIND THE MOTHERS IN YOUR

VILLAGE OR DISTRICT:

- *TO BREAST-FEED THEIR CHILDREN:*

  - *giving them nothing but mother's milk during the first four months*

  - *gradually adding other nourishing foods from the fifth month onwards*

- *NEVER TO FEED THE CHILD WITH FRESH OR TINNED MILK WHEN IT IS POSSIBLE TO BREAST-FEED*

- *NEVER TO USE A BOTTLE BUT INSTEAD A WELL-CLEANED CUP AND SPOON.*

ASK MOTHERS TO COME AND SHOW YOU THEIR BABIES EVERY MONTH TO HAVE THEM WEIGHED AND WHENEVER THEY ARE ILL.

WHEN THE BABY IS 5 MONTHS OLD

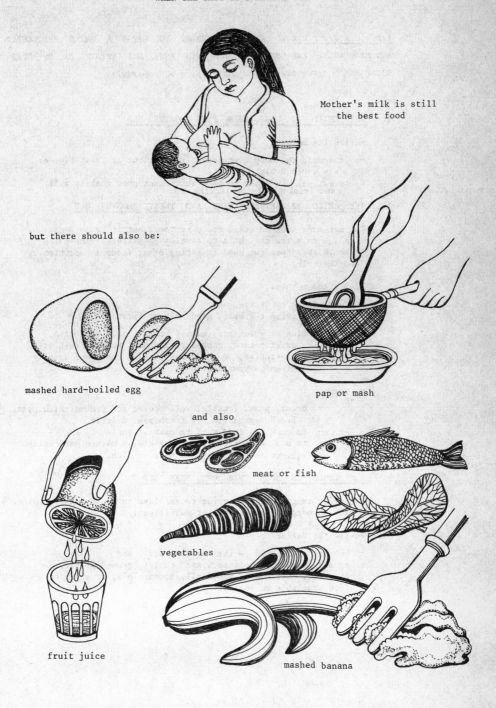

Mother's milk is still
the best food

but there should also be:

mashed hard-boiled egg

pap or mash

and also

meat or fish

fruit juice

vegetables

mashed banana

FEEDING THE CHILD

B E   C A R E F U L :   ALWAYS REMEMBER TO WEIGH A CHILD FREQUENTLY AND REGULARLY, AND SEE IF, FOR HIS AGE, HIS WEIGHT IS ON "THE RIGHT ROAD"   (see the growth chart, page 90 onwards)

1. <u>THE CHILD IS LESS THAN FIVE MONTHS OLD</u>

   Advise the mother:

   - to suckle the baby every time it asks, but at least five or six times a day
   - to eat well in order to have sufficient good quality milk and drink plenty of liquids

2. <u>THE CHILD IS BETWEEN FIVE AND TWELVE MONTHS OLD</u>

   The mother's milk is still the best food, but it is no longer enough to allow the child to develop completely. The child should therefore get used to eating other foods in addition to the milk.

   Advise the mother:

   - to continue to suckle, and
   - to start giving the baby, gradually at first:

     - rice or wheat pap, mashed banana, taro or potato, sweet potato, cooked groundnuts, mashed fruit or vegetables, or any other similar baby food usually given in your region

   - then:

     - beans, peas, lentils, well-cooked and ground chick peas, fresh vegetables and fresh peeled fruit
     - to cook the food well to make it easier to eat
     - to add, each time it is possible, a mashed hard-boiled egg, or some well-cooked meat or fish.

3. <u>THE CHILD IS MORE THAN ONE YEAR OLD</u>

   The child is gradually starting to eat like an adult and the mother's milk is becoming less and less sufficient.

   Advise the mother:

   - to watch her child so that he eats well, and
   - to add gradually foods such as: butter, groundnut oil, palm oil, cotton oil, wheat oil, coconut oil, or any other food available on the spot.

W H E N   Y O U   C A N

draw up

for each child

a

GROWTH CHART

based on the model on the two

following pages

You will be able to follow the growth of each child in your village/district by writing the weight down on the chart each time.

Your supervisor will give you the necessary instructions on how to use it and to decide which children should be referred for special care or supervision.

WHO 78066

GROWTH CHART

Health centre		Child's No.
Child's name		
Date first seen	Birthday	
Mother's name		Registration No.
Father's name		Registration No.
Where the family lives (address)		

BROTHERS AND SISTERS

Year/birth Boy/Girl	Remarks	Year/birth Boy/Girl	Remarks

IMMUNIZATIONS

ANTI-TUBERCULOSIS (BCG)

Date of immunization _____

WHOOPING COUGH, TETANUS AND DIPHTHERIA

Date of first injection _____
Date of second injection _____
Date of third injection _____

MEASLES

Date of immunization _____

SMALLPOX

Date of immunization _____
Date of scar inspection _____
Date of reimmunization _____

POLIOMYELITIS

Date of first immunization _____
Date of second immunization _____
Date of third immunization _____

APPOINTMENTS

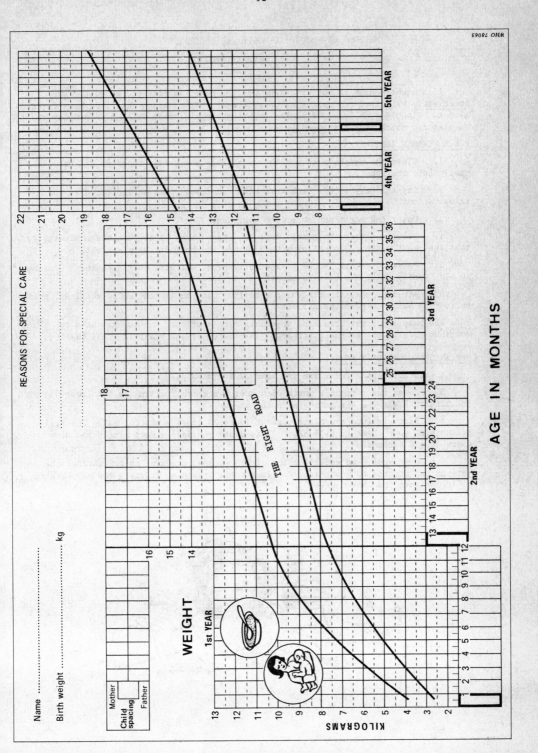

WHO 78065

METHOD OF MOUTH-TO-MOUTH RESUSCITATION

(Artificial Respiration)

If a newborn baby is not breathing but the heart is beating, he must immediately be helped to breathe or he will die. (The method described here is used also to help older children or adults to breathe again after falling into water or an electric shock, for instance.)

FOR A NEWBORN BABY:

1. Clean the mouth, nose and throat quickly and gently to allow air to pass easily into the chest.

2. Lay the baby on his back with his head tilted back as indicated in the illustration.

3. Cover the mouth and nose with your mouth.

4. Blow small breaths gently into the chest about 25 to 30 times a minute, so that the chest rises. Do not blow hard or you may harm the baby's chest.

5. Pause to see if he has started breathing, and blow gently again. Continue to blow gently until the baby is breathing regularly.

6. Air may pass into the child's belly. If you see the belly swell up, press on it from below to push the air out.

The baby may start breathing regularly almost at once, or you may have to continue to blow up his chest for about 15 minutes if the heart is still beating.

FOR AN OLDER CHILD OR ADULT:

1. and 2. Steps 1 and 2 are the same as for a baby.

3. Cover the patient's mouth with your own mouth, pulling up his lower jaw with one hand to clear the air passages to the chest.

4. Blow air into the patient about 15 to 20 times a minute, using the full pressure of your chest to fill his. This means you take a deep breath and blow every 3 or 4 seconds.

5. Lift your head and allow the air to escape, checking to see whether the patient has started to breathe. Continue until breathing starts: you may have to do it for more than one hour.

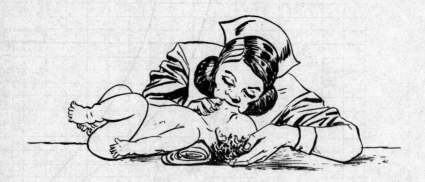

THE

BADLY - FED

CHILD

---

1. THE CHILD IS THINNER AND SMALLER THAN THE NORMAL CHILDREN OF HIS AGE

2. THE CHILD IS JUST SKIN AND BONE

3. THE CHILD'S FACE, LEGS, FEET AND (SOMETIMES) HANDS ARE SWOLLEN

THE BADLY-FED CHILD

LEARNING OBJECTIVES

At the end of training, the PHW should be able to:

1. Weigh a child

2. Decide whether the child has the right weight for
    his age

3. Recognize serious signs of malnutrition

4. Tell in what cases a child suffering from severe
    malnutrition should be sent to the hospital or
    health centre

DANGER

the child is just
skin and bone

his hair changes colour

DANGER

the child's face, legs
and feet are swollen

THE BADLY-FED CHILD

1. **EITHER THE CHILD IS THINNER AND SMALLER THAN THE HEALTHY CHILDREN OF HIS AGE**

   1.1 Ask how old the child is
   Weigh him and mark the corresponding place on the growth chart
   Look at the growth chart (page 91) to see if he is on "the right road"

   1.2 If he is not on the right road this child may be ill and he should be treated
   - has he got diarrhoea? See Problem 1.3, page 16
   - has he got a cough? does he have difficulty in breathing? See Problem 1.4, page 25
   - has he got worms? See Problem 6.6, page 185

   1.3 This child may not be well fed
   - ask the mother what he eats and see Problem 3.1, page 88, to advise the mother on what to give her child
   - see the child again after ten or fifteen days and weigh him;
     - if the child has put on weight and does not seem ill, tell the mother to continue feeding her child well
     - if not, send him to the hospital or the health centre

2. **OR THE CHILD IS JUST SKIN AND BONE**

   2.1 - he is very thin
   - his skin makes folds

   BE CAREFUL: it is serious, this child has not had enough to eat for a long time

   2.2 This child is perhaps ill and should be treated. See 1.2

   2.3 In any case, continue breastfeeding and start oral rehydration

   2.4 If the child vomits everything he eats, send him to the hospital or health centre at once.

3. **OR THE CHILD'S FACE, LEGS AND FEET ARE SWOLLEN**

   - he has no appetite, he has diarrhoea
   - the colour of his hair and skin is changing
   - he has no interest in his surroundings

   BE CAREFUL: it is serious, the child has not been eating what he should eat for a long time

   SEND HIM TO THE HOSPITAL OR THE HEALTH CENTRE IMMEDIATELY, if nothing can be done for him at home.

THE BADLY-FED CHILD

A child whose face, legs and feet are swollen, is a child who has been eating badly for a long time.

A child with a low birth weight, or not breast-fed, or exposed to infection may very quickly become just skin and bone.

You should prevent children from reaching this serious state by weighing the children in your community regularly and by following their growth on their "growth chart".

When growth is not on "the right road", see if the mother feeds her child well or if the child is ill.

It is by teaching mothers to feed their children well that the serious troubles of malnutrition will be avoided. See "Feeding the child" and talk to the mothers.

THE BADLY-FED CHILD

NEVER FORGET THAT MOTHER'S MILK IS BEST, FOR THE FOUR REASONS GIVEN ON PAGE 86.

However, it may happen that:

1.   The mother's breasts do not give enough milk

In this case advise the mother to drink plenty of water and other liquids and to eat well, including in her meals, if possible, peas, fresh vegetables, meat, milk and eggs.

She must drink a lot: the more water and other liquids she drinks and the better she eats the more milk she will have to feed her baby.

2.   The mother's breasts do not give any milk at all or the baby no
      longer has a mother to give him milk

In such cases the baby must be fed on other milk, either cow's or goat's milk or dried whole milk. Sweetened condensed milk and dried skim milk should only be used for feeding a baby if other milk is not available. Sweetened condensed milk contains too much sugar and too little milk, and skim milk too little fat; consequently, they are not sufficient for feeding a baby.

The preparation of milk for the baby from cow's or goat's milk and dried whole milk is long, difficult and can be dangerous if badly done:

- a correctly calculated amount of boiled water and sugar must
  always be added so as to have a milk just like mother's milk

- the baby must be weighed frequently so as to calculate the amount
  of milk it should take every day, since that amount depends on
  its weight

- the utensils necessary for preparing the milk (cup, spoon, etc.)
  should always be clean: otherwise the milk will contain germs
  which will make the baby ill

- cow's or goat's milk should always be boiled to kill any germs
  it may contain and so that the baby can digest it better

- as dried milk is expensive, it often happens that the person
  preparing the milk for the baby uses less dried milk than
  indicated, so that the milk thus prepared is inadequate and
  not sufficiently nourishing to ensure the baby's development.

CONSEQUENTLY, A MOTHER WHO HAS MILK SHOULD ALWAYS BREAST-FEED HER BABY. TELL AND ALWAYS REPEAT THIS TO ALL THOSE WOMEN WHO HAVE OR MAY HAVE CHILDREN. BUT WHENEVER A CHILD MUST BE FED ON MILK OTHER THAN MOTHER'S MILK CONSULT YOUR SUPERVISOR SO THAT HE CAN ADVISE ON THE BEST METHOD TO BE USED IN YOUR REGION.

B U R N S

BURNS ARE CAUSED BY FIRE, A RED-HOT OR BURNING
OBJECT AND ALSO BY BOILING WATER OR OIL.

THE SERIOUS THING IN A BURN IS THE AREA OF SKIN
IT COVERS.

BEFORE TREATING SOMEONE WHO HAS BEEN BURNT, WASH
YOUR HANDS CAREFULLY SO AS NOT TO DIRTY THE BURN.

LEARNING OBJECTIVES

At the end of his training, the PHW should be able to:

1. Tell whether the burn covers a small or a large
    area of skin

2. Tell when a patient with burns should be sent to
    the hospital or health centre

3. Tell whether the skin is covered with blisters only

4. Tell whether the skin is broken or has been removed

5. Clean a wound

6. Treat blisters and skin which is broken or has been
    removed

7. Treat a wound that smells bad or from which a
    yellowish fluid is coming out

8. Tell the patient and the family how to prevent burns

EACH AREA MARKED WITH *

= LARGE AREA

LARGE AREA

or

SMALL AREA

?

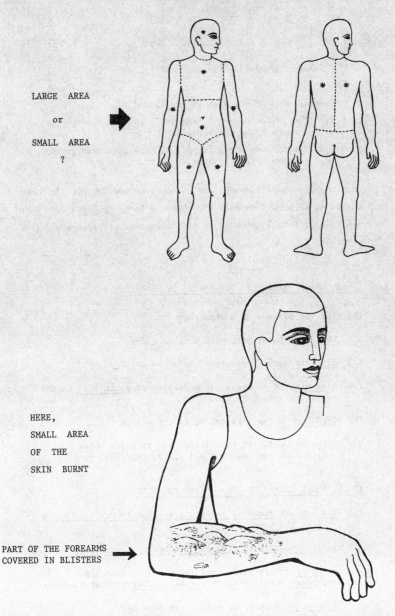

HERE,
SMALL AREA
OF THE
SKIN BURNT

PART OF THE FOREARMS
COVERED IN BLISTERS

B U R N S

Either

    1. A large area of the skin is burnt

or

    2. A small area of the skin is burnt, and

        2.1 The patient comes to see you less than twenty-four hours after the burn, or

        2.2 The patient comes to see you more than twenty-four hours after the burn.

When the burn covers as much as one arm, or one leg, or the head, or half the back, or more than half the chest, a large area has been burnt (see * of the drawing). When it is less than that, it is a small area of the skin.

1. IF A LARGE AREA OF THE SKIN IS BURNT

    1.1 Lay the patient on a stretcher

    1.2 Cover the burnt part with a clean cloth

    1.3 Give the patient plenty of water to drink

    1.4 Give him, if possible, an injection of penicillin in the buttock (see page 251)

    1.5 Send him to the hospital or health centre

    1.6 Show the people in the village how to avoid burns (see drawings, page 104, and 2.2.3, page 106)

2. IF A SMALL AREA OF THE SKIN IS BURNT

    2.1 The patient comes to see you less than twenty-four hours after the burn:

        2.1.1 The skin is covered with watery blisters only:

        - Wash gently with soapy water and a clean cloth
        - Cover with iodine or gentian violet without breaking the blisters
        - Put on a loose dressing (see drawing)
        - Tell the patient not to take the bandage off nor to dirty it

A SMALL AREA OF THE SKIN
IS BURNT

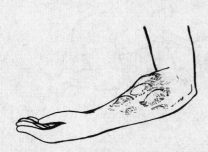

The skin is covered
with blisters

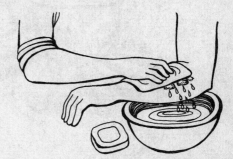

Wash gently with
soap and water

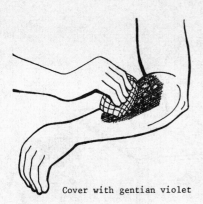

Cover with gentian violet

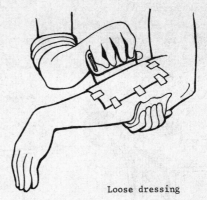

Loose dressing

BURNS

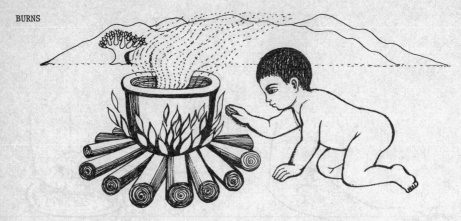

BE CAREFUL:

- <u>REMEMBER</u> THAT IT IS MAINLY CHILDREN WHO GET BURNT BECAUSE
  THEY DO NOT REALIZE THE DANGER:

    * A FIRE WITH NO GUARD ROUND IT

    * BOILING WATER

- <u>TEACH</u> PARENTS HOW THEY CAN PROTECT THEIR CHILDREN FROM THESE
  DANGERS

THEN YOU WILL HAVE FEWER BURNS TO TREAT.

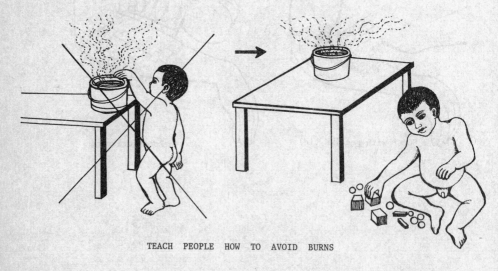

TEACH PEOPLE HOW TO AVOID BURNS

After a week take
off the bandage

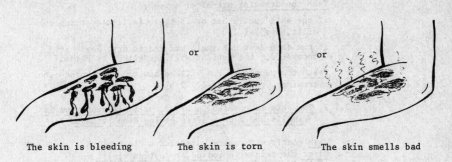

The skin is bleeding   or   The skin is torn   or   The skin smells bad

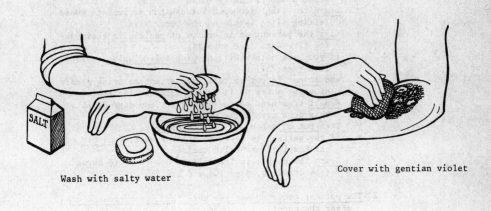

Wash with salty water   Cover with gentian violet

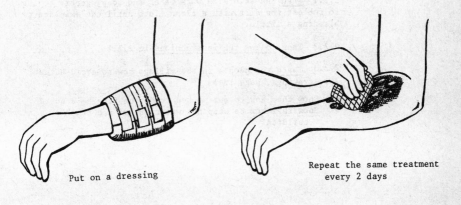

Put on a dressing   Repeat the same treatment
every 2 days

SALT

- <u>Take the dressing off</u> after a week:

  if the skin smells bad or if there is liquid coming out of it, see 2.1.2

  if the skin does not smell bad and is dry, leave it uncovered; the patient will get better by himself

- <u>Teach</u> the people in the village how to avoid burns (see drawings, page 104, and 2.2.3)

2.1.2 <u>The skin is covered in blood, or it is broken or it smells bad a week after having been bandaged</u>

- <u>Wash</u> gently with salty water and a clean cloth
- <u>Cover</u> the skin with <u>iodine</u> or <u>gentian violet</u>
- If it is an arm or a leg, <u>place</u> the burnt limb on a clean cloth soaked in salty water
- If it is another part of the body, <u>pat</u> with a clean cloth soaked in salty water
- <u>Leave</u> the skin uncovered but ask the patient to avoid letting flies settle on the burnt skin
- <u>Give</u> the patient an injection of <u>penicillin</u> every day for five days (see page 251)

  if you have no penicillin, <u>give</u> <u>sulfadiazine</u> tablets (see page 251)

  and <u>do not forget</u> to tell the patient to drink plenty of water while he is taking sulfadiazine tablets
- <u>Repeat</u> treatment of the skin every two days until a thin scab covers the wound
- Then <u>put on</u> a bandage (see drawing)
- If the patient is feverish after a week, <u>send him</u> to the hospital or health centre
- <u>Teach</u> the people in the village how to avoid burns (see drawings, page 104, and 2.2.3).

2.2 <u>The patient comes to see you more than twenty-four hours after the burn:</u>

2.2.1 <u>Wash</u> the skin with warm water and soap, gently trying to rub off the dirt with a clean cloth until the skin starts bleeding a little.

2.2.2 Then <u>follow the instructions</u> in 2.1.2

2.2.3 <u>Teach</u> the people in the village how to avoid burns (see drawings, page 104)

- <u>Show</u> them how to put stones round the fire as a guard
- <u>Show</u> them how to keep hot water out of the reach of children.

WOUNDS

THERE IS A WOUND WHEN THE SKIN IS CUT OR TORN.

A WOUND SHOULD BE CAREFULLY CLEANED AND THEN PROTECTED WITH A BANDAGE.

WOUNDS MAY ALSO MAKE THE PATIENT VERY TIRED AND WEAK; IN THAT CASE YOU SHOULD MAKE HIM DRINK AND SEND HIM TO THE NEAREST HOSPITAL OR HEALTH CENTRE.

LEARNING OBJECTIVES

At the end of his training, the PHW should be able to:

1. Stop blood flowing from a wound by pressing on the wound

2. Decide whether the flow of blood from a wound is very heavy or not

3. Recognize the major signs of extreme weakness

4. Decide when a wounded person should be sent to the hospital or health centre

5. Clean a wound, put disinfectant on it and put on a dressing

6. Bring the edges of a deep wound together in a straight line using either clips or sticking plaster

7. Watch over a patient who has had a heavy blow on the head, belly or chest

8. Put a bandage round a dressing

9. Tell a person with a wound what he must do when he goes home after treatment

10. Treat an old wound from which a yellowish fluid is coming out

11. Describe the three major signs of extreme weakness

12. Prepare and clean equipment

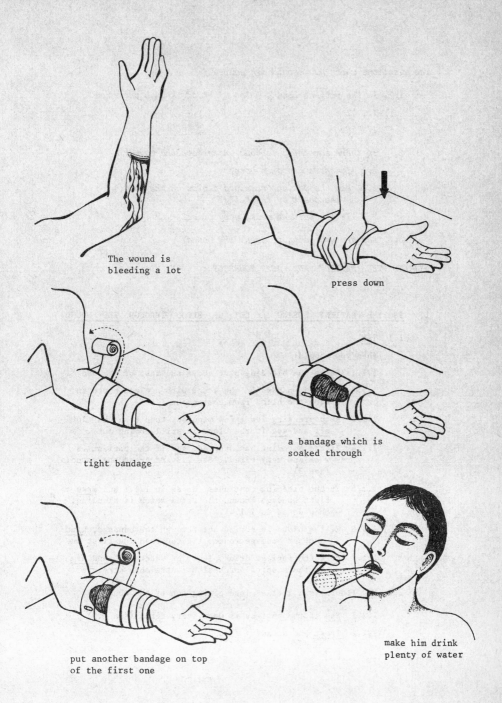

The wound is
bleeding a lot

press down

tight bandage

a bandage which is
soaked through

put another bandage on top
of the first one

make him drink
plenty of water

WOUNDS

The questions which you should ask yourself:

    1.   Is the patient losing a lot of blood through the wound?

        1.1 Yes

        1.2 No

    2.   Is there something serious underneath the wound?

        2.1 Is there a broken bone?

        2.2 Has the patient received a blow on the head, the chest or the belly?

        2.3 Is the patient weak, very tired?

    3.   How are you going to treat the wound?

EXAMINE THE PATIENT AND ASK YOURSELF :

1.   IS THE PATIENT LOSING A LOT OF BLOOD THROUGH THE WOUND?

    1.2 <u>Yes</u>

    Then you should:

    1.1.1 <u>Raise</u> the bleeding part above the rest of the body

    1.1.2 <u>Press down</u> hard on the wound with a clean cloth to stop the blood from coming out

    1.1.3 <u>Keep pressing</u> for a few minutes, then <u>take</u> the cloth <u>off</u> and <u>see</u> if the blood is still coming out

    1.1.4 If the bleeding has stopped, <u>see</u> if the patient is weak and very tired. See 2.3 and <u>treat</u> the wound(s) (see 3)

    1.1.5 If the bleeding continues, <u>do</u> as in 1.1.1 and <u>make</u> a tight bandage around the place which is bleeding; then <u>do</u> as in 1.1.4

    1.1.6 If the blood is coming out through the bandage, <u>wind</u> another bandage round, tighter than the first one

    1.1.7 <u>Make</u> the patient <u>drink</u> plenty of water and <u>send him</u> to the hospital or health centre on a stretcher.

    1.2 <u>No</u> (there is a little blood coming out of the wound(s))

    1.2.1 <u>See</u> if the patient is weak, very tired (See 2.3)

    1.2.2 <u>Treat</u> the wound(s) (See 3).

WOUNDS

2. IS THERE SOMETHING SERIOUS UNDERNEATH THE WOUND?

    2.1 Is there a broken bone?

    Yes: See Problem 4.3 "Fractures" (page 117)

    2.2 Has the patient received a blow on the head, the chest or the belly?

    Yes: Find out if the patient is feeling weak and tired

    If so, see Problem 6.7 (page 192)

    If not, treat the wound(s)
    see the patient again after three or four
    hours and then twice a day for the next
    two days. If the patient becomes very
    tired, send him to the hospital or health
    centre. If not, look after the wound(s).

    No: See 3

    2.3 Is the patient weak, very tired?

    2.3.1 Yes

    Then:

    - Make the patient drink plenty of water and send
    him to hospital or the health centre immediately
    - See Problem 6.7 "Weakness and tiredness".

    2.3.2 No

    Treat the wound(s). (See 3)

3. HOW TO TREAT THE WOUND

    3.1 It is a small wound

    3.1.1 Wash the wound with soap and water, using a compress
    (see No.1 of the drawing)

    3.1.2 Take off the dirt and shave off any hair all around
    the wound

    3.1.3 Put iodine or gentian violet on the wound and all
    around the wound (see No.2 of the drawing)

    3.1.4 Cover the wound completely with a clean piece of cloth
    and fasten the clean cloth with sticking plaster or
    string or cord or a piece of creeper (see No.3 and
    No.4 of the drawing)

    3.1.5 Tell the patient not to dirty the bandage nor to take
    it off

    3.1.6 Take the bandage off after five days

    3.1.7 If, when you take the bandage off on the sixth day, the
    wound smells bad, or there is liquid coming out of the
    wound, or the patient is feverish, see 3.2.6.

HOW TO CLEAN A WOUND:

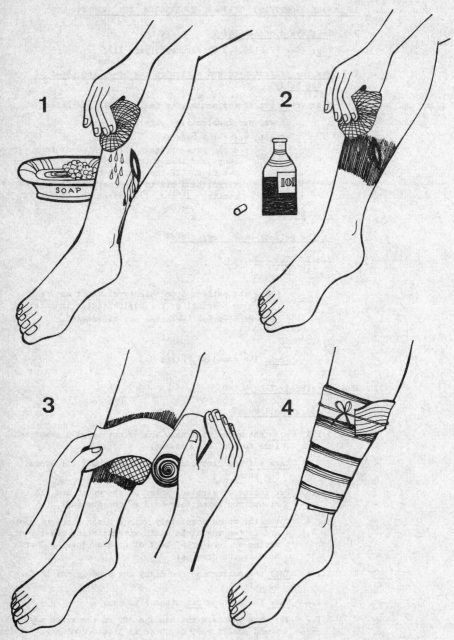

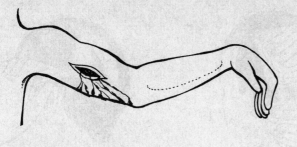

SMALL WOUND

SMALL DRESSING

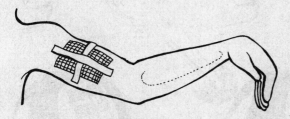

how to close a wound:

with

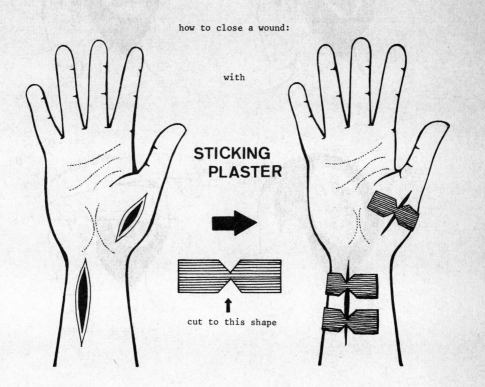

STICKING PLASTER

cut to this shape

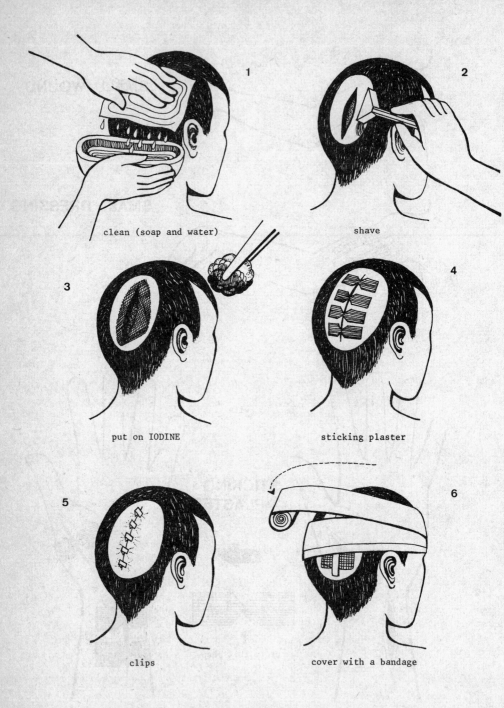

1 clean (soap and water)

2 shave

3 put on IODINE

4 sticking plaster

5 clips

6 cover with a bandage

3.2 **It is a large wound** (over 5 centimetres)

The patient should lie down or sit on a chair

3.2.1 **Wash** the wound with soap and water, using a compress

3.2.2 **Clean off** the dirt and **shave** off any hair around the wound

3.2.3 **Put** **iodine** or **gentian violet** on the wound and all around the wound

3.2.4 **Close up** the edges of the wound with sticking plaster (see drawing)

3.2.5 **Cover** the whole of the wound with a clean piece of cloth and fasten it with sticking plaster or string or cord or a piece of creeper, and ask the patient not to take the bandage off nor to dirty it

3.2.6 **Give** the patient one injection of **penicillin** every day for three days

- children: 500 000 units
- adults: 1 000 000 units

if you have no penicillin, give **sulfadiazine** tablets

- children: 1 tablet morning, noon and night for three days
- adults: 2 tablets four times a day for three days

3.2.7 **Take** the bandage **off** after five days:

1. The wound smells bad or liquid is coming out of the wound or the patient is feverish

- **Wash** the wound with salty water
- **Leave** it to dry and then **put** **iodine** or **gentian violet** on the wound and around the wound and **make a bandage** which you will change every two days
- **Give** an injection of **penicillin** or give **sulfadiazine** tablets as in 3.2.6
- **Do not forget** to change the bandage every two days
- If after a week the wound still smells bad or if liquid is still coming out of the wound, or if the patient is still feverish, **send** the patient to the hospital or health centre
- If not, **put** on a new bandage every five days until the wound is healed

2. The wound does not smell bad, there is no liquid coming out of the wound and the patient is not feverish

- **Cover** with **iodine** or **gentian violet**
- **Put** a bandage on and change it every five days until the wound has healed.

BE CAREFUL:

YOU SHOULD PREVENT ALL WOUNDS FROM LATER BECOMING WOUNDS

* WHICH SMELL BAD

* WHICH PRODUCE A YELLOWISH LIQUID

* WHICH MAKE THE PATIENT FEVERISH.

TO DO THIS,

- <u>WASH</u> YOUR HANDS CAREFULLY WITH SOAP BEFORE TOUCHING A WOUND

- <u>WASH</u> THE WOUND CAREFULLY BEFORE COVERING IT WITH A BANDAGE

- <u>WASH</u> YOUR HANDS AGAIN WHEN YOU HAVE PUT ON THE BANDAGE.

———

FRACTURES

WHEN A BONE IS BROKEN IT IS CALLED A FRACTURE.

YOU SHOULD PRESUME THERE IS PROBABLY A BROKEN BONE IF, AFTER A FALL OR A VIOLENT BLOW :

- THE PATIENT IS NOT ABLE TO MOVE THE LIMB

- IT HURTS A LOT WHEN THE PATIENT TRIES TO MOVE THE LIMB

- IT HURTS A LOT WHEN YOU PRESS YOUR HAND ON THE PART THAT HAS BEEN HIT

- THE LIMB IS OUT OF SHAPE.

FRACTURES

LEARNING OBJECTIVES

At the end of training, the PHW should be able to:

1. Find out from the patient
    - how the accident happened
    - where he feels pain

2. Examine a patient and tell if he can move his limbs, if he
   is breathing properly, and if he is fully conscious

3. Tell whether one of the patient's limbs (upper arm, forearm,
   hand, foot, lower leg or thigh) is out of shape

4. Decide whether a bone is broken by using both hands to feel
   a limb or move it gently

5. Straighten a broken bone by stretching the limb gently

6. Raise a limb in which the bone is broken and slide a flat
   length of wood (splint) under it

7. Put a bandage round the broken limb and the splint so that
   the limb cannot move

8. Tell what kind of fracture must be sent to the hospital or
   health centre

9. Tell how much time should pass before the patient should
   be seen again

10. Say what the patient or his family should be told to do
    before he is next seen

11. Give medicine or an injection as required

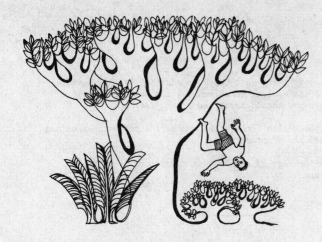

After
a fall
an accident
or a blow

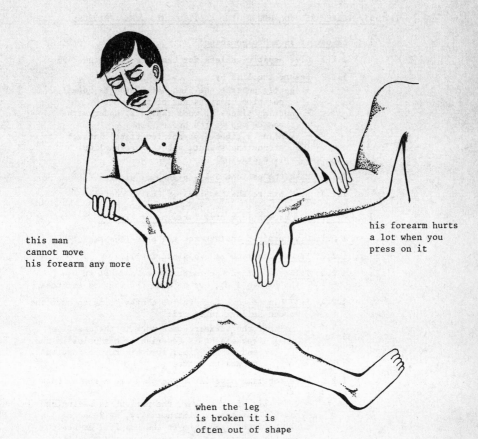

this man
cannot move
his forearm any more

his forearm hurts
a lot when you
press on it

when the leg
is broken it is
often out of shape

When you think the patient has a broken bone, you should:

1. *First see if there is a wound in addition to the fracture (cut or torn skin, sometimes you can see the bone), because you should treat the wound first;*

2. *Secure the broken limb before moving the patient, so as not to make the fracture worse;*

3. *Examine the rest of the body in case there is another fracture.*

———

1. IF THERE IS NO WOUND IN ADDITION TO THE FRACTURE

1.1 Either it is a broken thigh:

1.1.1 Give aspirin tablets for the pain (see page 249)

1.1.2 Secure the limb by:
- gently putting the limb back into its normal position if it is out of shape
- putting pieces of wood (splints) underneath and on top of the broken limb
- winding a tight (but not too tight) bandage around the splints and the broken limb (see drawing)

1.1.3 Make the patient drink plenty of water

1.1.4 Send him to the hospital or health centre

1.2 Or it is a broken leg, arm, forearm, or fingers

1.2.1 Give aspirin tablets for the pain (see page 249)

1.2.2 Secure the limb as explained in 1.1.2

1.2.3 Tell the patient to rest at home and not to use the broken limb, but to move the fingers and toes

1.2.4 Tell him to come back in two months' time to have the wooden splints taken off:
- if the patient comes back in the meantime because he is feverish or has pains in the end of the limb, send him to the hospital or health centre

1.2.5 Make the limb move after you have taken the splints off:
- if, after a week, the patient is beginning to use his limb normally, he is cured
- if not, send him to the hospital or health centre

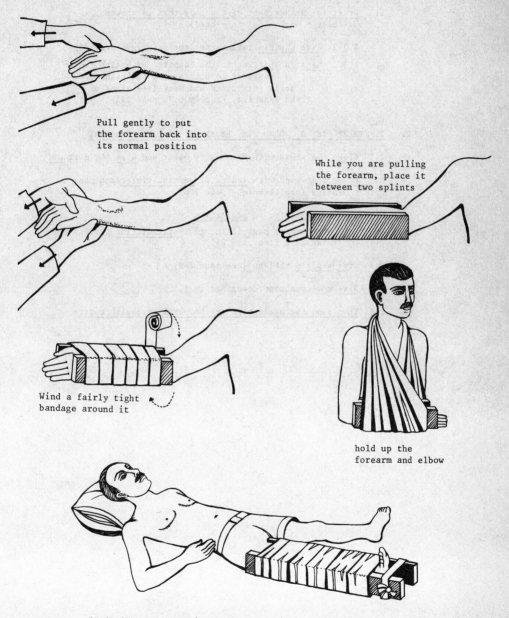

If the forearm
is broken

Pull gently to put
the forearm back into
its normal position

While you are pulling
the forearm, place it
between two splints

Wind a fairly tight
bandage around it

hold up the
forearm and elbow

if it is a broken thigh or leg,
do it this way

1.3 <u>Or it is another part of the body that is broken</u>
(chest - back - pelvis - head)

    1.3.1 <u>Give aspirin</u> tablets for the pain (see page 249)

    1.3.2 <u>Send</u> the patient to the hospital or health centre
if he continues to complain of bad pains, or
if he is very tired and weak (see signs of
great weakness, Problem 6.7, page 192)

2. <u>IF THERE IS A WOUND IN ADDITION TO THE FRACTURE</u>

2.1 <u>Clean</u> the wound with warm salty water and <u>wipe</u> the dirt <u>off</u>

2.2 <u>Cover</u> the wound with <u>iodine</u> or <u>gentian violet</u> and make a
bandage (see technique page 250)

2.3 <u>Give an injection</u> of <u>penicillin</u>

    If you have no penicillin, give <u>sulfadiazine</u> tablets for
three days (see page 251)

2.4 <u>Give aspirin</u> tablets (see page 249)

2.5 <u>Give</u> the treatment described in 1.1.2

2.6 <u>Then send the patient to the hospital or health centre.</u>

BITES

YOU CAN BE BITTEN BY A DOG OR BY A SNAKE. A SNAKE-BITE IS ALWAYS DANGEROUS: THE PATIENT SHOULD BE TREATED AS QUICKLY AS POSSIBLE.

A DOG-BITE IS ONLY DANGEROUS IF THE DOG IS BEHAVING IN A STRANGE WAY.

YOU SHOULD TREAT ANY OTHER KIND OF BITE AS YOU WOULD TREAT A WOUND.

BITES

LEARNING OBJECTIVES

At the end of his training, the PHW should be able to:

1. Treat the wound caused by a dog-bite

2. List four strange signs in a dog's behaviour

3. Find out whether the dog which has bitten is known or not

4. Decide whether the dog was behaving in a strange way

5. Describe the signs when a person bitten by a dog should be sent to the hospital or health centre

6. Treat a person who has been bitten by a snake

7. Describe the usual treatment given by the villagers

8. Organize group discussions in the village to discuss snake-bites and dog-bites

THE PATIENT HAS BEEN BITTEN:

- EITHER BY A DOG

- OR BY A SNAKE

---

1. **IF THE PATIENT HAS BEEN BITTEN BY A DOG**

   1.1 **First of all look after the person who has been bitten**

   1.1.1 **Clean** the wound with soap and water

   1.1.2 Then **cover** the wound with **iodine**

   1.1.3 **Put** a bandage on

   1.1.4 **Never close** the wound with sticking plaster

   1.2 **Ask if someone knows the dog that bit the patient**

   1.2.1 **Someone knows the dog:**
   it is the family dog or a neighbour's dog

   Ask if the dog's behaviour had changed

   - if it had stopped eating
   - if it barked in an unusual way
   - if it trembled, was savage, never stopped barking
   - if it had convulsions (fits), if saliva ran out of its mouth

   If it showed any of these symptoms, then **have** the dog **killed** and **send** the person who has been bitten to the hospital or health centre immediately.

   If the dog had not shown any of these symptoms

   Ask for the dog to be watched for ten days

   If during that time it begins to show any of these symptoms, then **have** the dog **killed** and **send** the person who has been bitten to the hospital or health centre immediately. If the dog stays healthy, you need do nothing else.

   1.2.2 **No one knows the dog that bit the patient:**
   it is a dog which does not belong to the village

   In this case, **send** the person who has been bitten to the hospital or health centre.

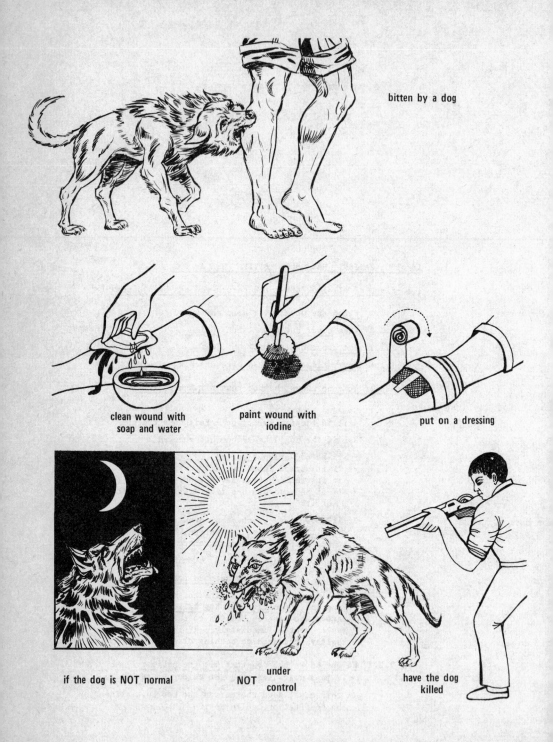

bitten by a dog

clean wound with
soap and water

paint wound with
iodine

put on a dressing

if the dog is NOT normal

NOT under
control

have the dog
killed

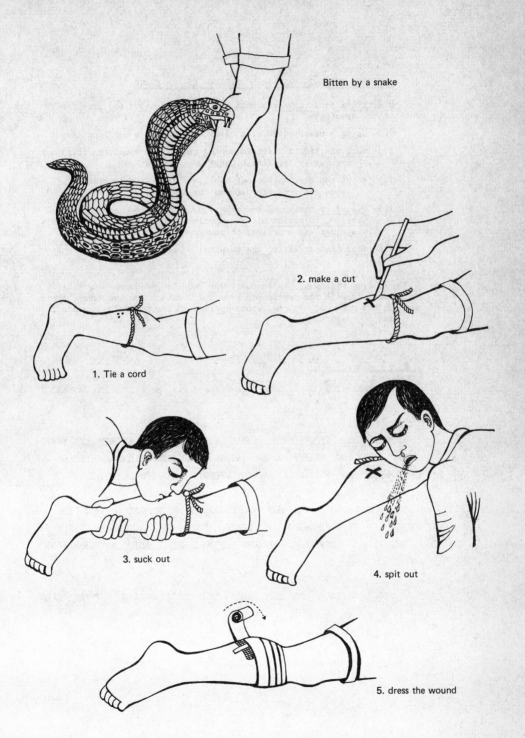

Bitten by a snake

1. Tie a cord

2. make a cut

3. suck out

4. spit out

5. dress the wound

BITES

2. IF THE PATIENT HAS BEEN BITTEN BY A SNAKE

    2.1 Tie a cord tightly around the limb just above the bite (see
         drawing)

    2.2 Using a razor-blade or a clean knife, make a cut 1 cm deep

    2.3 Suck the liquid which is coming out of the wound, spitting out
         immediately the liquid which you have sucked

    2.4 After you have sucked out the liquid for 5 to 10 minutes,
         loosen the cord tied around the limb

    2.5 Disinfect the wound and make a bandage
         Give an injection of one ampoule of antivenom (medicine
         against snake poison) if you have some

    2.6 Send the patient to the hospital or health centre.

N.B. In some villages, people sometimes know how to cure snake-bites.
Talk about it with the people who know. If you have no antivenom, their
methods may work well (porous stone applied to the bite, for example).

BE CAREFUL :

    A SNAKE-BITE OR A DOG-BITE (see 1.2.1, page 125) IS DANGEROUS
AND MAY CAUSE DEATH.

    SICK DOGS OFTEN BITE PEOPLE AND ANIMALS. DO NOT GO NEAR
THEM. ALL DOGS THAT WANDER AROUND THE COUNTRYSIDE MAY BE
DANGEROUS. DO NOT WALK AROUND WITHOUT CARRYING A STICK.

    EXPLAIN TO PEOPLE HOW TO RECOGNIZE SICK DOGS. TELL THE
PEOPLE IN THE VILLAGES AND THEIR CHIEFS IF SOMEONE HAS BEEN
BITTEN BY A SICK DOG, BECAUSE IT MAY BITE OTHER PEOPLE LATER
ON.

    TEACH CHILDREN TO KEEP AWAY FROM SICK DOGS AND FROM SNAKES.

WATER SUPPLY

DIRT CAUSES DISEASE. IF YOU WASH WITH CLEAN WATER AND SOAP THE DIRT ON YOUR BODY WILL COME OFF. YOU SHOULD DRINK ONLY CLEAN WATER SO THAT DIRT WILL NOT GET INSIDE YOUR BODY.

IF YOU WANT TO BE HEALTHY, FIND ALL THE WAYS OF GETTING AS MUCH CLEAN WATER AS POSSIBLE.

TO HAVE CLEAN WATER, EITHER TAKE WATER FROM A PROTECTED SPRING OR WELL OR BOIL ANY OTHER WATER BEFORE YOU DRINK IT.

WATER SUPPLY

<u>LEARNING OBJECTIVES</u>

At the end of his training, the PHW should be able to:

1. Find the place where villagers go to get water for
    drinking and for washing themselves

2. Tell which pond or river water can be safe for
    drinking

3. Recognize whether water from a spring or well is
    safe for drinking

4. Explain to the people the danger of drinking
    dirty water

5. Show the people how they can get clean water
    from a spring or well

The water in a POND

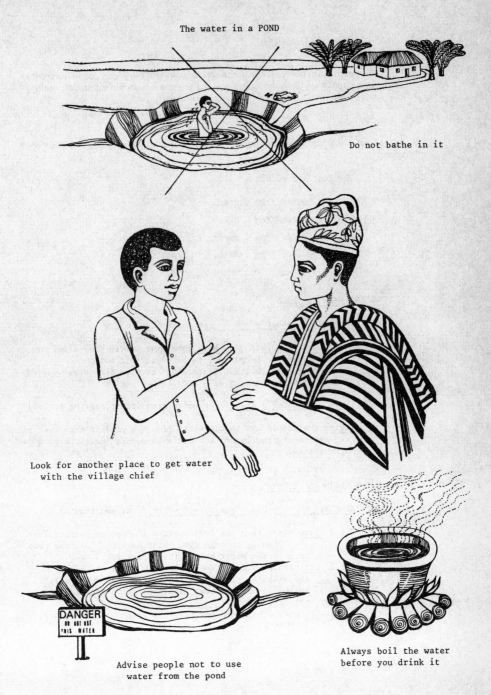

Do not bathe in it

Look for another place to get water
with the village chief

Advise people not to use
water from the pond

Always boil the water
before you drink it

DANGER
DO NOT USE
THIS WATER

WATER SUPPLY

> *The people in the village have asked you how they can get clean water, or your supervisor has asked what you have done about this problem since his last visit.*

> W H A T   D O   Y O U   D O ?

See where the people get the water they use and decide on what action to take.

> *The people use:*

> 1. *water from a pond*
> 2. *water from a river*
> 3. *water from a spring*
> 4. *water from a well.*

1. WATER FROM A POND

1.1 There is no other place to get water from

1.1.1 Tell the people to boil the water before they drink it
1.1.2 Advise the people not to bathe in this water
1.1.3 Discuss with the village chief to find some other way of getting water (see 3 and 4)

1.2 There is another place to get water from (river, spring or well)

Advise the people not to use water from the pond if the other place to get water from is not too far away and to leave the pond for the cattle.

2. WATER FROM A RIVER

2.1 If there is no other place to get water from, you should:

2.1.2 Draw water from the river before it reaches your village (see drawing on page 133, point No 1). Tell the people to boil the water before they drink it
2.1.2 Let people bathe in the river only where it leaves the village; let the animals drink the water only further down the river (see drawing on page 133, points 2 and 3)
2.1.3 Let people bathe in the river if your supervisor says they may.

2.2 There is a spring or a well

See 3 or 4.

WATER from a RIVER

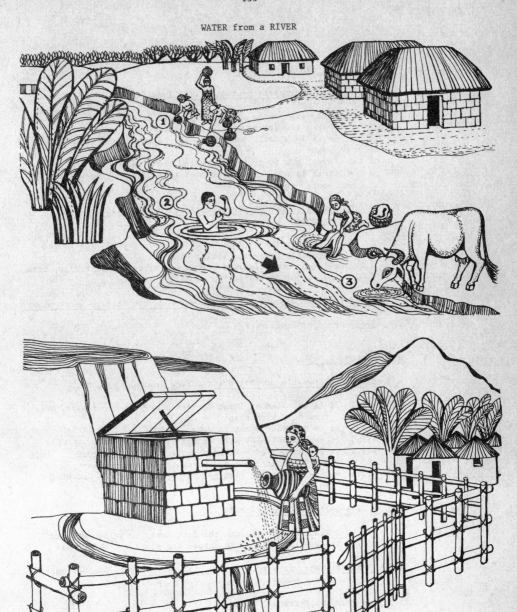

A properly protected SPRING

3. WATER FROM A SPRING

    3.1 The spring is properly protected if: (see drawing)

        3.1.1 There is a fence all the way round it about 20 metres away
            from the spring, and the gate is kept closed
        3.1.2 There is a ditch around the spring to let the rainwater drain
            away
        3.1.3 There is a 50 cm high cemented stone wall round the spring
        3.1.4 There is a pipe coming out of this wall and the water is
            taken from this pipe

    3.2 If the spring is not properly protected or if no spring
       is being used

        3.2.1 Go and see the village chief and help the village to get
            properly protected spring water
        3.2.2 See your supervisor if you cannot arrange to get water from
            a spring or protect it properly

    3.3 If the village wants to bring the water to the village along pipes

    See your supervisor.

4. WATER FROM A WELL

    4.1 A well is properly protected if: (see drawing, page 135)

        4.1.1 It is situated at least 20 metres away from a latrine or
            from a rubbish heap
        4.1.2 It is at least 3 metres deep
        4.1.3 It is lined inside with stones stuck with mortar
        4.1.4 It is surrounded by a stone wall which is about 50 cm high
        4.1.5 There is a ditch for the rainwater to drain away
        4.1.6 People do not let dirt get into it and they do not wash
            in it

    4.2 If the well is not protected:

        4.2.1 Go and see the village chief to have the well protected
        4.2.2 See your supervisor to choose the place for a new well

    4.3 If the village wants to make the well work better (by putting in
       a lever or a pump):

    See your supervisor.

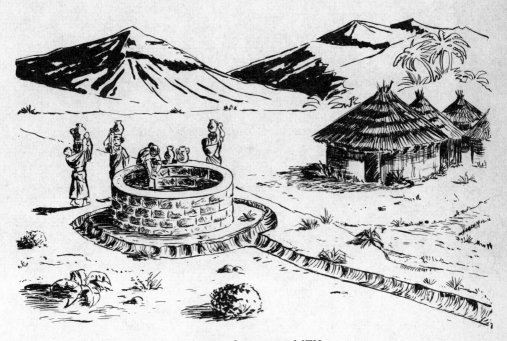

A properly protected WELL

EXCRETA

DISPOSAL

PEOPLE SHOULD NOT DEFECATE JUST ANYWHERE, BECAUSE FAECES
CARRY DISEASES.

PEOPLE SHOULD DEFECATE ONLY IN PLACES WHERE NEITHER THEY,
NOR CHILDREN, NOR ANIMALS, NOR FLIES CAN TOUCH THE FAECES.

EXCRETA DISPOSAL

LEARNING   OBJECTIVES

At the end of his training, the PHW should be able to:

1. Find out the places where the village people go to
    defecate

2. Explain that it is dangerous to defecate just
    anywhere

3. Give advice on why and how to build a latrine

4. Decide whether or not a latrine is being properly
    used

5. Teach people how to use a latrine properly

EXCRETA DISPOSAL

The people in the village have asked you about having a good place for defecating or your supervisor has asked you what you have done, since his last visit, to improve the situation.

W H A T   A R E   Y O U   G O I N G   T O   D O ?

See where the villagers go to defecate and <u>*decide*</u> *what action to take.*

1. *The people use a latrine*

2. *The people defecate around the house*

3. *The people defecate in the river*

4. *The people defecate in the fields or in the forest.*

1. THE PEOPLE USE A LATRINE

   1.1 <u>To be properly used a latrine should:</u>

      1.1.1 Be built at least twenty metres away from a house, a river, a well or a spring

      1.1.2 Have the hole at least one metre deep

      1.1.3 Have the hole covered with a slab (made of wood or concrete) which has a hole in the middle

      1.1.4 Have the hole in the middle of the slab covered with a lid

      1.1.5 Be covered by a roof and surrounded by a wall made of branches

   1.2 <u>If the latrine is not being properly used</u>

      1.2.1 <u>Give</u> advice to the head of the family

      1.2.2 <u>See</u> if there are any faeces on the slab. If so, <u>have it cleaned</u> with water

      1.2.3 Go and <u>have a look</u> now and then to see if the people are following your advice.

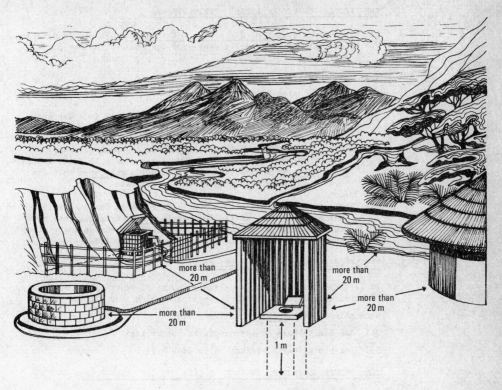

A PROPERLY BUILT LATRINE

the slab over the latrine
must be kept clean

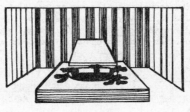

DANGER
clean with water
frequently

EXCRETA DISPOSAL

2. THE PEOPLE DEFECATE AROUND THEIR HOUSES

2.1 There is a danger of disease from the faeces when people defecate less than twenty metres away from the house or on the paths which lead to the house

2.1.1 Advise the heads of families

- either to tell their families to defecate in the fields (see 4)
- or to tell their families to defecate in a latrine (see 1)

2.1.2 See the village chief and ask him to speak to the people in the village. If he wants the people to build latrines, see your supervisor and afterwards make sure that the latrines are being properly used (see 1.1)

2.2 There is less danger if the people defecate as far as possible from houses. However, advise the people not to defecate less than twenty metres away from the houses, see the advice to be given when people defecate in the fields or in the forest (see 4).

3. THE PEOPLE DEFECATE IN THE RIVER

It is dangerous when people defecate in the river or less than twenty metres away from the river or on a path which leads to the river.

When this happens, see the village chief:

3.1 Ask him to talk to the people in the village

3.2 Ask him to have latrines built (see 1.1).

4. THE PEOPLE DEFECATE IN THE FIELDS OR IN THE FOREST

4.1 There is little danger of disease if people defecate in the fields or in the forest provided that they do it:

4.1.1 More than twenty metres away from a house, a spring, a river or a well

4.1.2 Far away from a path or a track

4.2 If the animals usually eat in the field where the people go to defecate, see your supervisor and the village chief
In any case, advise the people to defecate in a little ditch and to cover their faeces with some earth.

BE CAREFUL:

TO AVOID THE DISEASES CARRIED BY FAECES,

DEFECATE

1. IN A LATRINE

2. OR ELSE IN A HOLE FAR AWAY FROM THE HOUSE, AND THEN COVER THE FAECES WITH EARTH

3. AND ALWAYS FAR AWAY FROM THE RIVER, A WELL, A SPRING OR A PATH

WHAT YOU SHOULD NOT DO:

WHY ?

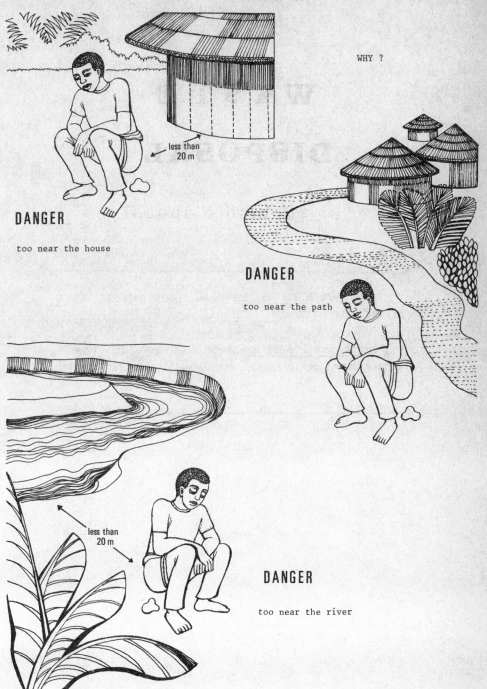

less than
20 m

DANGER

too near the house

DANGER

too near the path

less than
20 m

DANGER

too near the river

WASTE

DISPOSAL

(or, rubbish disposal)

WASTE SHOULD NOT BE THROWN AWAY JUST ANYWHERE, BECAUSE IT MAY CARRY DISEASE.

PEOPLE SHOULD THEREFORE THROW WASTE IN PLACES WHERE NEITHER THEY, NOR CHILDREN, NOR ANIMALS, NOR FLIES CAN TOUCH IT.

WASTE DISPOSAL

LEARNING OBJECTIVES

At the end of his training, the PHW should be able to:

1. Find out the places where the village people
    generally go to throw their waste

2. Decide whether the village pit is being properly
    used or not

3. Explain to the village chief how the village pit
    should be used

4. Decide whether or not waste is being properly thrown
    away outside houses

5. Explain to the head of a family how to throw away
    waste properly outside a house

6. Decide whether or not it is dangerous to throw away
    waste in the fields (or in the forest)

7. Get in touch with his supervisor and ask him to
    come and help the villagers with his advice

WHAT YOU <u>SHOULD</u> <u>NOT</u> DO

Do not throw wastes:

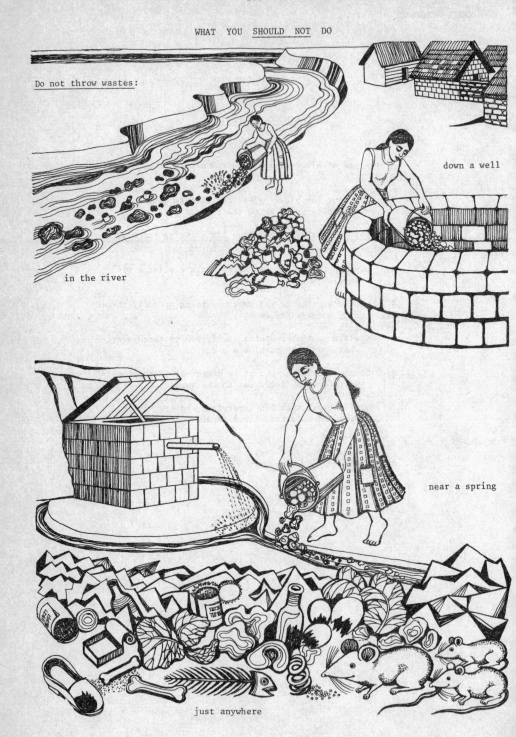

down a well

in the river

near a spring

just anywhere

WASTE DISPOSAL

> *The people in the village have asked you about having a good place in which to throw their waste, or your supervisor has asked what you have done since his last visit to make sure that the people have a good place in which to throw their waste.*
>
> *W H A T   A R E   Y O U   G O I N G   T O   D O ?*
>
> *See where the people go to throw their waste and decide what action to take.*
>
> 1. *The people throw their waste into a common pit*
>
> 2. *The people throw their waste outside their houses*
>
> 3. *The people throw their waste near the river*
>
> 4. *The people throw their waste in the fields.*

1. THE PEOPLE THROW THEIR WASTE INTO A COMMON PIT

   1.1 To be properly used the pit should:

   1.1.1 Be outside the village and about twenty metres away from a house

   1.1.2 Be in a hollow and not on top of a hill

   1.1.3 Be at least 100 metres away from a river, a well or a spring

   1.1.4 Have the waste piled up in a hole and not scattered around

   1.1.5 Have the waste covered with a layer of earth which is two to three centimetres thick

   1.1.6 Be surrounded by a fence made of branches

   1.2 If the pit is not being properly used:

   1.2.1 Explain to and show the village chief how to get a good common pit (see 1.1)

   1.2.2 See if your advice is being properly followed by visiting it regularly.

WHAT YOU CAN DO WITH WASTE

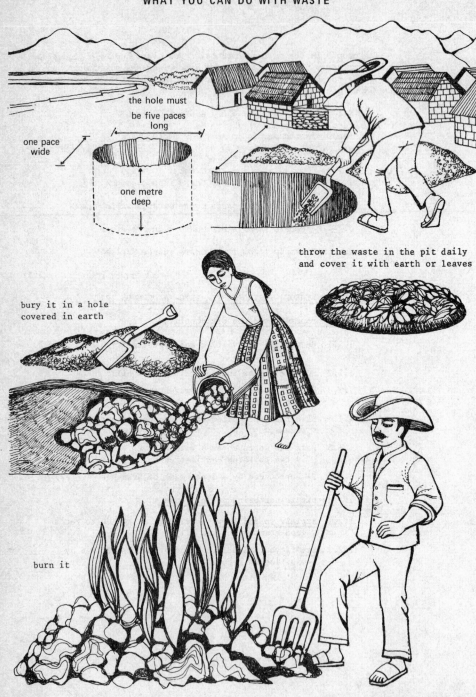

the hole must be five paces long

one pace wide

one metre deep

throw the waste in the pit daily and cover it with earth or leaves

bury it in a hole covered in earth

burn it

WASTE DISPOSAL

2. <u>THE PEOPLE THROW THEIR WASTE OUTSIDE THEIR HOUSES</u>

    2.1 <u>Waste is being properly disposed of when:</u>

        2.1.1 It is piled up in a hole and not scattered around

        2.1.2 It is put at least twenty metres away from a house,
    a river, a spring or a well

        2.1.3 It is covered with a little earth to stop animals
    and flies from coming to it and eating it

    2.2 <u>If it is not properly disposed of:</u>

        2.2.1 <u>Explain to</u> and <u>show</u> the head of the family how to
    dispose of waste outside his house (see drawing)

        2.2.2 <u>Advise</u> the village chief to have a common pit dug

        2.2.3 <u>Ask</u> your supervisor to come and help in having the
    pit dug

        2.2.4 <u>See</u> if the new pit is being properly used (see 1.1)

3. <u>THE PEOPLE THROW THEIR WASTE NEAR THE RIVER</u>

    3.1 <u>See</u> the village chief (2.2.2)

    3.2 <u>See</u> the head of the family (2.2.1)

4. <u>THE PEOPLE THROW THEIR WASTE IN THE FIELDS</u>

    4.1 There is little danger provided the waste is not piled up
    less than 100 metres away from the house, a river, a well
    or a spring

    4.2 If it is thrown less than 100 metres away:
    <u>See</u> the village chief (2.2.2)
    <u>See</u> the head of the family (2.2.1).

B E   C A R E F U L :

   * *TO AVOID THE DISEASES CARRIED BY WASTE*

              <u>GET RID OF IT</u>

*1. IN A HOLE FAR AWAY FROM YOUR HOUSE AND FROM THE
WATER WHICH THE PEOPLE DRINK*

2. OR BY BURNING IT ONCE A WEEK.

   * *IF YOU USE A SEPARATE HOLE FOR THE WASTE WHICH COMES
FROM PLANTS (LEAVES, VEGETABLES, FRUIT, ROOTS), YOU
WILL SOON HAVE <u>FERTILIZER</u> FOR GROWING MORE VEGETABLES
AND OTHER PLANTS.*

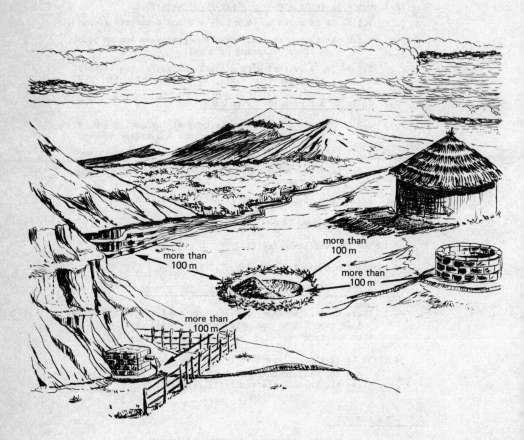

A WELL - SITUATED COMMON PIT

FOOD

PROTECTION

FOOD IS VERY PRECIOUS; THEREFORE :

- YOU SHOULD NOT WASTE IT OR LET IT GO BAD

- YOU SHOULD KEEP IT CLEAN

FOOD PROTECTION

LEARNING OBJECTIVES

At the end of his training, the PHW should be able to:

1. Find out what kinds of food the village people eat

2. List four ways to store grain to protect it from rats

3. List three precautions to take when buying food from
     a trader

4. Demonstrate to the housewife how to store food in
     the house

5. Show how hands should be washed

6. Show how to cook food, by boiling, etc.

7. Show how to put food on a clean plate

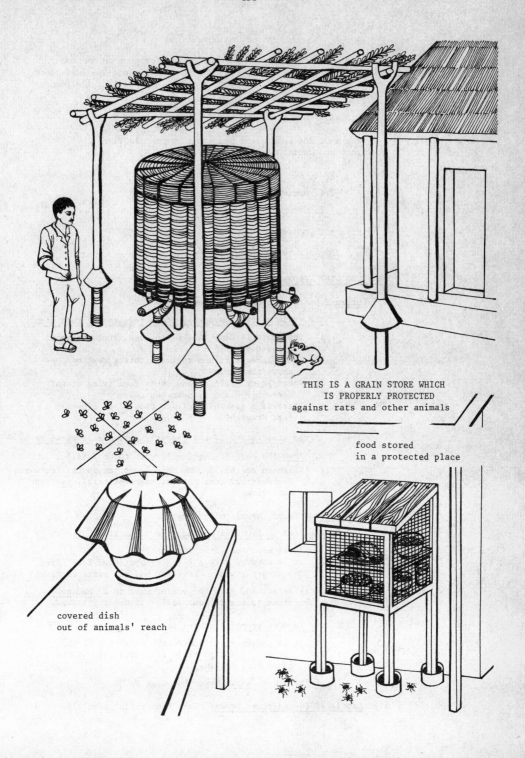

THIS IS A GRAIN STORE WHICH
IS PROPERLY PROTECTED
against rats and other animals

food stored
in a protected place

covered dish
out of animals' reach

FOOD PROTECTION

*There are at least five new patients with diarrhoea in one week,
or your supervisor has asked you what you have done since his last visit
to have the village food protected, or you have noticed that the food
was stored carelessly.*

W H A T   A R E   Y O U   G O I N G   T O   D O ?

*See what the people eat and how they prepare their
food and decide what action to take.*

1. WHAT DO THE PEOPLE EAT ?

1.1 Grain

1.2 Other foods

2. HOW DO THEY PREPARE THEIR FOOD ?

3. HOW DO THEY STORE THEIR FOOD ?

1. <u>WHAT DO THE PEOPLE EAT</u> ?

1.1 <u>Grain</u> (wheat, or rice, or millet ...)

1.1.1 <u>The grain store is properly protected against rats if</u>:

1. The grain is kept in a place that is closed in on
    all sides
2. This place is raised at least thirty centimetres
    above the ground
3. There is no grain or any other food lying around
    near this place or near the house
4. There is a lid which closes this place properly
    (see drawing)

1.1.2 <u>If the grain store is not properly protected against rats</u>:

1. <u>Show</u> the head of the family what to do (see 1.1.1)
2. If there are still some rats about one month afterwards
    (someone has seen rats or signs of rats), <u>see</u> your
    supervisor

1.2 <u>Other foods</u> (meat, bread, milk, eggs ...)

1.2.1 <u>The food bought from a trader is clean if</u>:

1. It is kept away from the sun
2. It is covered with a cloth or protected from flies
3. The trader's hands are clean and his place is clean

If it is not so, <u>show</u> the trader what to do and <u>come</u>
sometimes to see if your advice is being followed

1.2.2 <u>The food is properly stored in the house if</u>:

1. It is put in a container covered with a cloth
2. It is put in a high place in a cool part of the
    house (see drawing)

If it is not, <u>show</u> the mother what to do

1.3 <u>Little grain and other foods</u>: See "Foodstuffs" page 224.

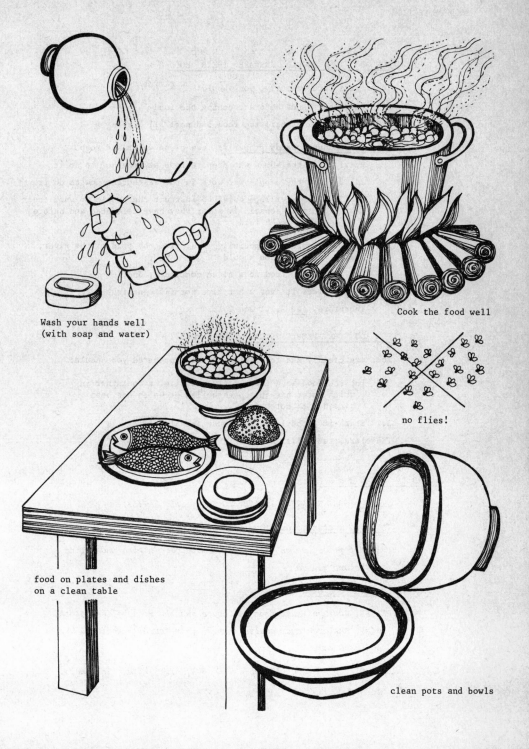

Wash your hands well
(with soap and water)

Cook the food well

no flies!

food on plates and dishes
on a clean table

clean pots and bowls

FOOD PROTECTION

2. <u>HOW DO THE PEOPLE PREPARE THEIR FOOD</u> ?

To prepare food properly, you should:

2.1 Wash your hands before touching the food

2.2 Either cook or boil the food and peel <u>all</u> fruits

2.1 <u>To wash your hands properly</u>: use clean water and soap

    2.1.1 <u>Show</u> the women who prepare food at home how to do it

    2.1.2 <u>Show</u> the people who work in the restaurant how to do it

    2.1.3 <u>Ask</u> the village chief to instruct the people to wash their hands, especially after they have defecated and before they touch food

2.2 <u>To boil the food</u> (especially water from the pond or the river, milk and meat) you should:

    2.2.1 Put the food in a clean container, and

    2.2.2 Place it over a hot fire for fifteen minutes

Therefore, <u>see</u> 2.1.1 and 2.1.2

3. <u>HOW DO THE PEOPLE STORE THEIR FOOD</u> ?

To store cleanly the food which has been prepared you should:

3.1 Put the food in a clean container, i.e. a container in which water has just been boiled or which has been rinsed with hot water

3.2 Store it properly in the house (see 1.2.2)

Therefore, see 2.1.1 and 2.1.2.

BE CAREFUL :

DIRTY FOOD BRINGS DISEASE TO ALL THE FAMILY.

* <u>*To avoid wasting clean food:*</u>

PREVENT flies, worms, rats and animals from coming and eating it before you do

* <u>*To keep food clean:*</u>

PREVENT things (dust from the house and the road, flies, cloth, mice, children's or adults' hands) from touching what you are going to eat.

PROTECT YOUR FOOD AGAINST THE SUN, THE WIND, THE RAIN.

SKIN
DISEASES

PEOPLE WHO HAVE SKIN DISEASES BUT NO OTHER SIGNS OF
SICKNESS SHOULD WASH THEIR SKIN, COVER IT WITH A MEDICINE
AND KEEP THEIR HANDS VERY CLEAN.

PEOPLE WHO HAVE A HIGH TEMPERATURE AS WELL AS A SKIN
DISEASE SHOULD BE GIVEN A MEDICINE TO BE TAKEN BY MOUTH
OR TO BE INJECTED INTO THE BUTTOCKS, AND ANOTHER MEDICINE TO
PUT ON THE SKIN.

SKIN DISEASES

LEARNING OBJECTIVES

At the end of his training, the PHW should be able to:

1. Find out whether an accident has been the cause of
    the skin problem

2. Decide whether the skin disorder covers a small or
    large area

3. Recognize when there is a lump (or a swelling) under
    the skin

4. Tell if the skin is covered with red <u>spots</u> or red
    <u>patches</u> or <u>blisters</u> or <u>scabs</u>

5. Treat a patient who has fever and has red spots
    covering a large area of skin

6. Treat a patient who has fever and has blisters and
    scabs over a large area of skin

7. Tell whether a patient has been scratching the skin

8. Treat a patient who scratches when there are no scabs

9. Treat a patient who scratches when a large area of the
    skin is covered with scabs

10. Treat a patient who scratches a small area of his skin

11. Treat a patient whose skin is covered with small scabs
    that have fluid coming out from under them

12. Decide when a patient with a skin problem should be
    sent to the hospital or health centre

13. Talk with village people about how to prevent skin
    problems

SKIN DISEASES

How did the skin disease start?

1. After an accident?

2. Not after an accident?

    2.1 The patient is feverish
        2.1.1 a small area of the skin is affected
        2.1.2 a large area of the skin is affected
    2.2 The patient is not feverish
        2.2.1 it itches
        2.2.2 it does not itch.

1. <u>IT IS AFTER AN ACCIDENT</u>

    See Problems: 4.1 "Burns"

                  4.2 "Wounds"

                  4.3 "Fractures".

2. <u>IT IS NOT AN ACCIDENT</u>

    Take the patient's temperature (see page 252)

    Either the patient is feverish
    Or the patient is not feverish.

- 158 -

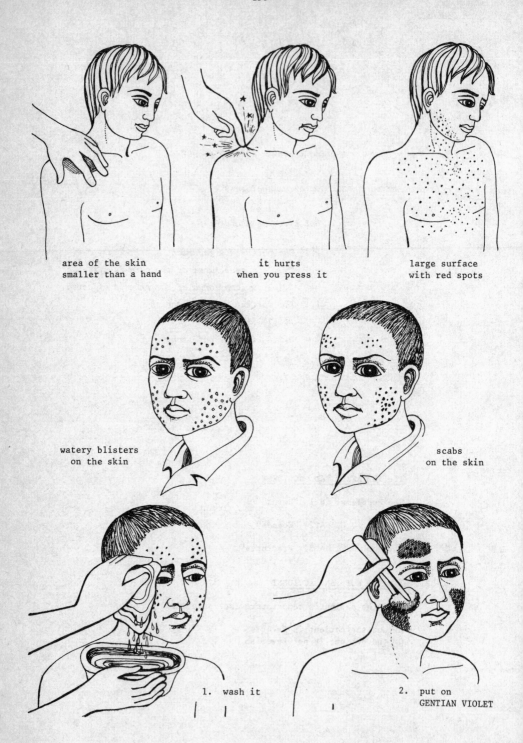

area of the skin
smaller than a hand

it hurts
when you press it

large surface
with red spots

watery blisters
on the skin

scabs
on the skin

1. wash it

2. put on
GENTIAN VIOLET

SKIN DISEASES

2.1 The patient is feverish

2.1.1 A small area of the skin is affected

1. If it is a lump which feels hot and which hurts when
   you press it with your finger, see Problem 6.9
   "Lumps under the skin"

2. If it is something else, put on compresses of salty
   water three times a day (one tablespoon of salt into
   one litre of water). Give sulfadiazine tablets for
   three days,

   children under 3 years: 1 tablet morning, noon and night
   children over 3 years: 2 tablets morning and night
   adults: 2 tablets morning, noon and night

   Always drink plenty of water with sulfadiazine

2.1.2 A large area of the skin is affected (more than the size of a hand)

1. There are red spots or patches

   - Give an injection of penicillin every day for three
     days

     children: 500 000 units
     adults: 1 000 000 units

     If you have no penicillin, give sulfadiazine tablets
     as stated above

   - See the patient again on the fourth day:
       If he is no longer feverish, the patient is
         getting better
       If he is still feverish, send the patient to the
         hospital or health centre

2. There are watery blisters or scabs, see drawing

   - Wash the skin with soap and water

   - Then put gentian violet on the skin

   - Give penicillin or sulfadiazine as stated above

   - See the patient again on the fourth day:
       If he is still feverish, send him to the hospital
         or health centre
       If he is no longer feverish, the patient is getting
         better

3. There is a large wound. See Problem 4.2 "Wounds".

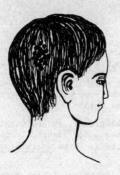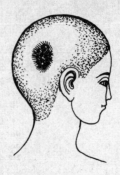

you should shave the hair on the head
before you treat the scalp

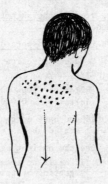

scabs

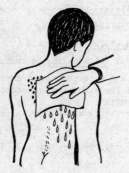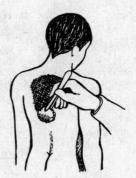

1. wash them

2. put on
GENTIAN VIOLET

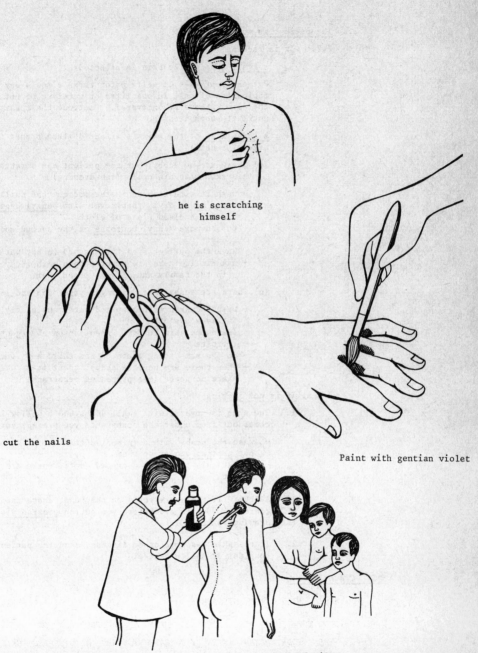

he is scratching
himself

cut the nails

Paint with gentian violet

treat the whole family

SKIN DISEASES

2.2 The patient is not feverish

2.2.1 It is itching

1. A small area of the skin is affected:

   Put on compresses of salty water three times a day (one tablespoon of salt in one litre of water). Do not wipe the skin. Leave it uncovered. Continue the treatment until it stops itching.

2. A large area of the skin is affected (larger than the size of a hand)

   (a) There are no scabs, but the patient has scratched his skin with his nails (see drawing)

   - wash it with soap and water and cut the nails
   - leave it to dry; then cover with benzyl benzoate, using a clean piece of cloth
   - put on more benzyl benzoate on the second and third day
   - have the patient's clothes washed in hot water
   - ask him if there are other people with itchy skin in the family and, if so, treat them.

   (b) There are scabs (see drawings, pages 158 and 160)

   - wash the skin with soap and water and gently try to take scabs off
   - leave the skin to dry; then put on some gentian violet
   - do the same thing again on the third and fourth day
   - when there are no more scabs, treat it as when there are no scabs (see preceding paragraph)

2.2.2 It is not itching

1. The skin is covered with small scabs and a yellow liquid comes out from under the scabs when you press them:

   - wash the scabs with soap and water
   - put gentian violet on them
   - repeat this treatment every day until there are no scabs left.

   BE CAREFUL: If there are scabs on the head, shave the hair off before you wash it and before you put on gentian violet (see drawing, page 160).

2. If the skin has some other disease, send the patient to the hospital or health centre.

BE CAREFUL:

TO AVOID MANY SKIN DISEASES:

1. DO NOT TOUCH THE DISEASED SKIN OF ANOTHER PERSON
2. WASH YOUR HANDS AFTER YOU HAVE TOUCHED A DISEASED SKIN
3. IF A MEMBER OF YOUR FAMILY HAS A SKIN DISEASE, GET HIM TREATED

EYE

DISEASES

YOU USUALLY CATCH EYE DISEASES:

- BECAUSE YOU RUB YOUR EYES WITH <u>DIRTY HANDS</u> (AFTER WORKING WHERE THERE IS EARTH OR DUST, WHEN YOU HAVE A RUNNY NOSE, WHEN YOU HAVE TOUCHED A WOUND OR A DISEASED SKIN)

- BECAUSE YOU DO NOT PROTECT YOUR EYES WHEN YOU ARE <u>WORKING IN DANGEROUS CONDITIONS</u> (WHEN YOU ARE CUTTING WOOD, WHEN YOU ARE BREAKING STONES, WHEN YOU ARE HARVESTING ...)

- BECAUSE YOU ARE NOT EATING WELL.

DO NOT FORGET TO WASH YOUR HANDS <u>BEFORE</u> AND <u>AFTER</u> TOUCHING THE EYES.

EYE DISEASES

<u>LEARNING OBJECTIVES</u>

At the end of his training, the PHW should be able to:

1. Show the village people how to protect themselves
    against eye diseases

2. Treat a child or adult whose eyes are running

3. Put ointment in the eyes of a baby a few days
    old who has runny eyes

4. Treat the baby's father and mother with penicillin
    injection

5. Treat a child or adult who has one or both eyes
    running

6. Send to the hospital or health centre any patient:

    -   who can no longer see out of one or both eyes
    -   who has pain in one or both eyes
    -   who has got something in his eye
    -   whose eyes continue to run even after treatment

EYE DISEASES

IF YOU WANT TO PROTECT THE PEOPLE LIVING IN YOUR

VILLAGE AGAINST EYE DISEASES, ADVISE:

- *the people to wash their faces and hands with soap and water after working, when they have a runny nose, when they have touched a wound or a diseased skin, and to come and see you when they have an eye disease,*

- *the people who help to deliver babies to clean the eyes of a new-born baby carefully,*

- *the mothers to feed their children well and tell them that carrots fruit and green vegetables are good food to eat for the eyes,*

- *the teachers to show the schoolchildren how to wash their faces and hands with soap and water and to send any child who cannot see properly to the doctor or community nurse.*

WHEN YOU SEE SOMEONE WITH AN EYE DISEASE, CARRY OUT THE

FOLLOWING INSTRUCTIONS:

IF, ON WAKING UP,
THE EYELIDS ARE STUCK TOGETHER BY DISCHARGE AND DIRT
YOU SHOULD CLEAN THE EYELIDS WITH A DAMP CLOTH
AND THEN OPEN THEM TO ENABLE THE EYE TO SEE

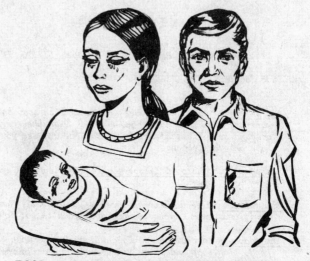

PUS RUNS FROM BABY'S EYES
HE IS SICK....MOTHER AND FATHER TOO

(but they may not know it!)

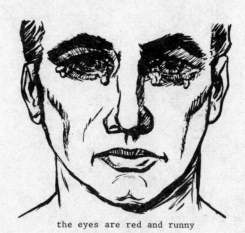

the eyes are red and runny

EYE DISEASES

1. IF THE PATIENT CAN NO LONGER SEE PROPERLY WITH ONE OR
   BOTH EYES

   This may be serious.

   Send the patient to the hospital or health centre.

2. IF ONE EYE HURTS

   This may be caused by, for example, some dust, a splinter, a little
   piece of straw ...

   The patient complains that one eye hurts and that it is red and
   runny.

   Wash your hands well with soap and water and look underneath the
   eyelids of the eye that hurts (see drawing).

   If you see a little dust, a small fly or something else on the
   eyelid, take the corner of a clean piece of cloth and rub very gently
   to remove it.

   - Rinse the eye with clean water

   - Then put on some aureomycin ointment (see page 249) or tetracycline
     ointment (see page 251) and ask the patient to come back and see
     you the following day:

     - if the eye no longer hurts, put on some more aureomycin
       ointment and tell the patient to come back and see you
       if the eye starts hurting again

     - if the patient's eye still hurts, send him to the hospital
       or health centre.

   If you cannot see anything underneath the eyelids, send the patient to
   the hospital or health centre.

HOW TO FOLD THE EYELID BACK TO REMOVE
SOMETHING FROM THE EYE

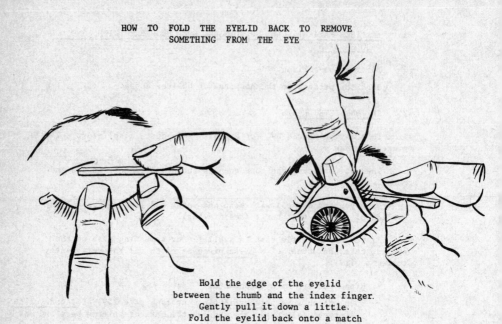

Hold the edge of the eyelid
between the thumb and the index finger.
Gently pull it down a little.
Fold the eyelid back onto a match
held in the other hand.

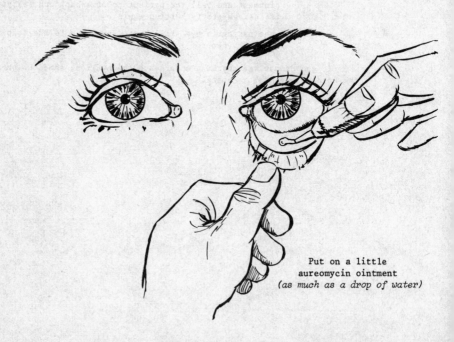

Put on a little
aureomycin ointment
(as much as a drop of water)

EYE DISEASES

**3.   IF ONE OR BOTH EYES ARE RUNNY, BUT THE PATIENT SEES WELL
AND THE EYES DO NOT HURT**

3.1   If the patient is a baby a few days old

A lot of pus is running out of one or both eyes

BE CAREFUL: This is a disease which the baby caught while he was
being born because his mother and father are ill and perhaps other
members of the family,too. You should therefore treat both the
baby and the parents, and any brothers and sisters as well.

For the baby: put a little aureomycin eye ointment in each eye three
times a day for five days, having first cleaned the eyelids with a
damp cloth, or ask the parents to do so.
If you have no eye ointment, send the baby to the hospital or
health centre immediately.

For the father and mother: you should give them both an injection
of 4 000 000 units of penicillin in the buttock, and give them
the same injection again the following day.
If you have no penicillin, send them both to the hospital or
health centre.

See both the baby and his parents again after four or five days.

Either everything is all right: they are cured
Or they are no better: send them to the hospital or health centre.

3.2   If the patient is a child or an adult

A discharge like water or milk is running out of one or both eyes.

Tell the patient:

-   to put warm damp compresses on the eyelid(s)

-   to put aureomycin eye ointment in both eyes every morning and
    night for five days, and

-   to wash the hands well several times a day with soap and water.

There is no more discharge from the eye(s): the patient is cured.
There is still discharge from the eye(s): send the patient to the
hospital or health centre.

HEADACHES

PEOPLE HAVE HEADACHES FOR MANY REASONS.

WHEN IT IS NOT SERIOUS, THE HEADACHE GOES AWAY BY ITSELF OR WITH THE HELP OF ASPIRIN.

WHEN IT IS SERIOUS, YOU SHOULD SEND THE PATIENT TO THE HOSPITAL OR HEALTH CENTRE.

LEARNING OBJECTIVES

At the end of training, the PHW should be able to:

1. Treat a patient with headache but no other signs
    of illness

2. Examine a patient with headache

3. Demonstrate how to know if a patient has a
    stiff neck

4. List four things about the behaviour of a patient
    that shows he is behaving in a strange way

5. Decide when to send a patient to the hospital or
    health centre

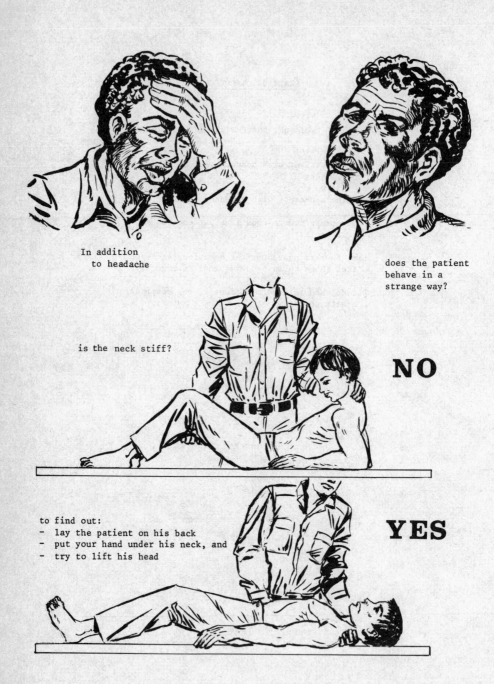

In addition
to headache

does the patient
behave in a
strange way?

is the neck stiff?

NO

to find out:
- lay the patient on his back
- put your hand under his neck, and
- try to lift his head

YES

HEADACHES

EITHER

1. <u>THE HEADACHE IS NOT SERIOUS</u>:

   - it goes away by itself
   - it goes away with the help of some <u>aspirin</u> (see page 249)

OR

2. <u>THE HEADACHE IS SERIOUS</u>:

   - it does not go away with the help of aspirin

   IN ADDITION TO HEADACHE

   2.1 The patient <u>has fever</u>. See Problem 1.2

   2.2 The patient's <u>neck is stiff</u>

   The neck is stiff when a patient, who is either standing or
      lying down with his legs stretched out, cannot touch his
      chest with his chin by himself, or if you cannot easily
      move his head to do the same thing (see drawing)

   <u>Send</u> the patient to the hospital or health centre.

   2.3 The patient is <u>behaving in a strange or odd way</u>

   The patient seems very lost and does not know where he is,
      or he does not answer when you ask him questions,
      or he tells stories which are not true,
      or he talks or walks like someone who has drunk too much alcohol

   <u>Send</u> the patient to the hospital or health centre.

   2.4 The patient has <u>swollen legs and feet</u>

   <u>Send</u> him to the hospital or health centre.

Problem 6.4
BELLY PAINS

BELLY PAINS

    TO HAVE BELLY PAINS IS TO HAVE PAINS EITHER ALL OVER THE BELLY OR IN A PART OF IT.

BELLY PAINS

At the end of his training, the PHW should be able to:

1. List three conditions that cause pain in the belly

2. Give medicine to a patient with sudden and severe
    pain in the belly

3. Give medicine to a patient with <u>recurrent</u> pains
    in the belly

4. Give advice to a patient with pains in the belly

5. Treat a patient with pains in the lower belly

6. Treat a patient with fever and pain in the belly

7. Send to the hospital or health centre any patient:
    - who still has pain in the belly after
        treatment
    - who has severe pain with vomiting

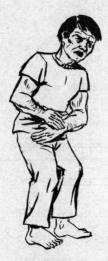

Very bad pain
in the belly

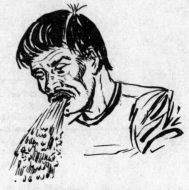

has he vomited?
has he **diarrhoea**?
has he got worms?

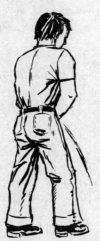

has he
pain in the
lower belly
when urinating?

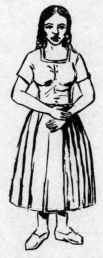

if a woman,
has she got her period?

BELLY PAINS

When a patient comes to see you because of belly pains, you should ask if the pain is very bad or not:

1. <u>IS THE PAIN VERY BAD</u> ?

The pain came on in a few minutes or in a few hours, the patient has very bad belly pains and has difficulty in walking.

    1.1 It is the <u>first time</u> that the patient has felt this particular pain.
Give the patient an injection of <u>atropine</u> or give him some drops of <u>belladonna</u> (see technique, page 249)
Tell the patient not to eat or drink anything and send him to the hospital or health centre immediately.

    1.2 It is <u>not the first time</u> that the patient has felt this particular pain.
Give the patient an injection of <u>atropine</u> or give him some drops of <u>belladonna</u> (see technique, page 249) and make him lie down for two hours.
See the patient again after two hours:
If the pain goes, let the patient go home and tell him to come back if the pain starts again. If the pain starts again, send the patient to the hospital or health centre.
If the pain continues, send the patient to the hospital or health centre.

2. <u>IS THE PAIN NOT VERY BAD</u> ?

    2.1 The patient has <u>diarrhoea</u>:
See "Diarrhoea" page 16.

    2.2 The patient has <u>worms in his stools</u>:
See "Intestinal worms" page 185.

    2.3 The patient has <u>not got diarrhoea or worms in his stools</u>

        2.3.1 The patient has mild pains in the belly <u>after he has eaten</u>:
Tell the patient to eat slowly and not to work immediately after eating
Ask the patient not to eat fatty foods (fried food, cakes, pork meat)
Give him some drops of <u>belladonna</u> (see technique, page 249).
See the patient again after two weeks:
If he is better, tell him to stop taking the drops of <u>belladonna</u> but to continue to eat slowly and to avoid fatty foods.
If he is no better, send him to the hospital or health centre.

BELLY PAINS

2.3.2 The patient has <u>pains in the lower belly or when he urinates</u>

Take his temperature:

(a) the patient is <u>not feverish</u>

Give him <u>aspirin</u> (see page 249)
Tell him to drink plenty of liquid
See him again after three days.
   If he is all right, he is cured. Advise him
     to drink more liquid than usual.
   If he is no better, send him to the hospital
     or health centre;

(b) the patient <u>is feverish</u>

Give the patient <u>sulfadiazine</u> tablets (see page 251)
See the patient again after five days:
   If he is all right, the patient is cured. Advise
     him to drink more liquid than usual
   If he is no better, send him to the hospital or
     health centre.

3. <u>THE PATIENT IS A WOMAN WHO HAS PAINS IN THE BELLY EVERY TIME SHE HAS A PERIOD</u>

See Problem 2.5 "Diseases of women" page 79.

———

PAINS IN THE JOINTS

PAINS IN THE JOINTS ARE COMMON.

WHEN THESE PAINS START AFTER AN ACCIDENT OR A FALL OR AFTER AN INFECTION, THEY SHOULD BE TREATED IMMEDIATELY SO THAT THE PATIENT CAN GO BACK TO HIS NORMAL OCCUPATION.

WHEN THESE PAINS OCCUR IN OLD PEOPLE WHO HAVE NOT HAD AN ACCIDENT AND WHO DO NOT HAVE AN INFECTION, THE PAIN SHOULD BE TREATED, BUT YOU SHOULD ALSO KNOW THAT THESE PAINS WILL COME BACK: THIS IS A DISEASE OF OLD AGE. IN THOSE CASES, ASPIRIN IS THE BEST MEDICINE.

PAINS IN THE JOINTS

LEARNING OBJECTIVES

At the end of his training, the PHW should be able to:

1. Tell whether pain in a joint is due to a fracture
    or to a wound

2. Put a tight bandage round a painful joint

3. Explain to a patient how he should rest after pain
    caused by an accident

4. List three signs of infection in a joint

5. Decide whether or not there is heat in a joint

6. Decide whether or not a joint has changed shape

7. Treat a patient who is feverish and has pain in a
    joint

8. Decide when a patient with a painful joint should
    be sent to the hospital or health centre.

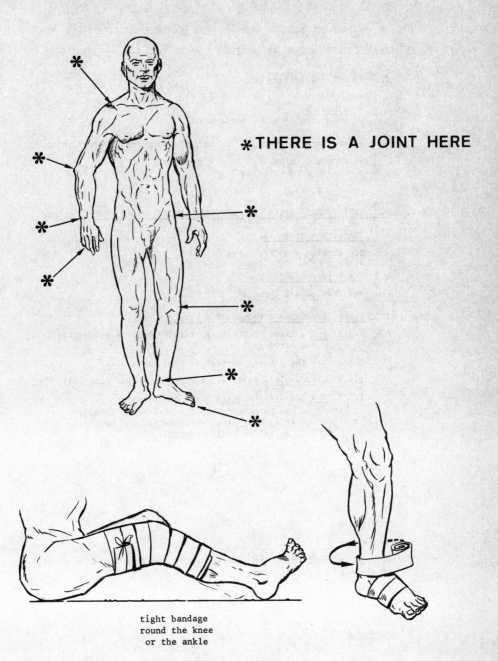

*THERE IS A JOINT HERE

tight bandage
round the knee
or the ankle

IF A PATIENT HAS A PAIN IN ONE OR MORE JOINTS, ASK HIM IF THEY STARTED AFTER AN ACCIDENT OR A FALL ?

1. *If so, has he also got:*
   - *a fracture*
   - *a wound*
   - *neither a fracture nor a wound*

2. *If not, has he also got, in addition to pains in the joints:*
   - *signs of infection*
   - *no signs of infection*

1. <u>DID THEY START AFTER AN ACCIDENT OR A FALL? YES</u>

   1.1 <u>There is a fracture</u>

   See Problem 4.3 "Fractures"

   1.2 <u>There is a wound</u>

   See Problem 4.2 "Wounds"

   1.3 <u>There is neither a wound nor a fracture</u>

   1.3.1 <u>Put</u> a tight (but not too tight[1]) bandage around the joint (see drawing)

   1.3.2 <u>Ask</u> the patient to rest at home for a week

   1.3.3 <u>Give aspirin</u> tablets for three days (see page 249)

   1.3.4 <u>See</u> the patient <u>again</u> after one week:
   - he has no more pain: the patient is cured
   - he still has pain: send the patient to the hospital or health centre.

---

[1] A bandage is too tight if it causes pain or swelling below the joint, in the fingers or the toes.

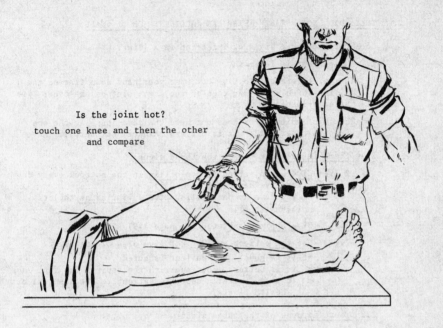

Is the joint hot?
touch one knee and then the other
and compare

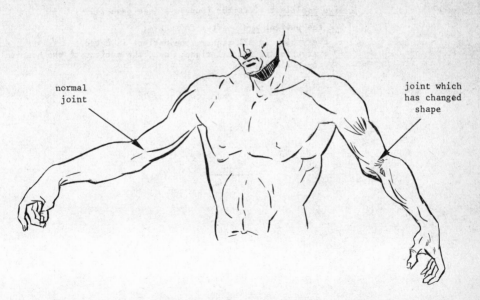

normal
joint

joint which
has changed
shape

PAINS IN THE JOINTS

2. THEY DID NOT START AFTER AN ACCIDENT OR A FALL

Look for the three signs of infection in a joint:

1. The patient is feverish

2. The joint is hot. To find out, put your hand down flat on the
   joint which hurts and then on the same joint on the other limb
   (see drawing)

3. The joint which hurts does not have the same shape as the one
   on the other limb: it is bigger, thinner, stiffer ...

2.1 There is at least one of the three signs

2.1.1 Give an injection of penicillin in the buttock every day
for five days (see page 251)
If you have no penicillin, give sulfadiazine tablets
(see page 251)

2.1.2 Give aspirin tablets (see page 249)

2.1.3 See the patient again after five days of treatment:
   - it is gone: the patient is cured
   - it is better: continue with the aspirin for five days
   - it is no better: send the patient to the hospital or
     health centre.

2.2 There is none of the three signs

Give aspirin tablets for four days (see page 249)

See the patient again after four days:
- everything is all right: the patient is cured
- everything is not all right: send the patient to the hospital
  or health centre.

INTESTINAL

WORMS

WORMS MAY BE FOUND IN FOOD IN ALL COUNTRIES. THEY
ENTER THE BODY WITH THE FOOD AND THEN LIVE IN THE PATIENT'S
INTESTINE. THEY LIVE ON THE FOOD WHICH THE PATIENT EATS AND
MAKE HIM TIRED.

THE WORMS LAY EGGS WHICH COME OUT OF THE BODY IN THE
STOOLS.

WHEN A PATIENT HAS WORMS IN THE INTESTINE AND HE LEAVES
HIS STOOLS ON THE GROUND - AND NOT IN A LATRINE - THE WORMS'
EGGS WILL SPREAD EVERYWHERE AND GET INTO THE WATER WE DRINK
AND THE FOOD WE EAT. THIS IS HOW WORMS PASS FROM ONE
PATIENT TO ANOTHER.

TO FIGHT AGAINST THESE WORMS YOU SHOULD CARRY OUT THE
FOLLOWING INSTRUCTIONS.

INTESTINAL WORMS

LEARNING OBJECTIVES

At the end of his training, the PHW should be able to:

1. Tell village people three ways to prevent them from getting worms

2. Recognize the three main types of intestinal worms

3. Treat a patient who is passing or vomiting roundworms or flatworms

4. Treat a patient who complains of itching around the anus at night

5. Treat the other members of the patient's family if necessary

6. Send to the hospital or health centre any child who:
    - vomits and passes worms
    - has severe pain in the belly accompanied by vomiting.

YOU CATCH INTESTINAL WORMS

- *because you eat with <u>dirty hands</u> (you have not washed them after using the latrine, after working or playing on the ground)*

- *because you eat <u>fruit</u> which has <u>fallen on the ground</u> where there are eggs from intestinal worms, without washing that fruit first*

- *because you eat <u>beef or pork which is raw or not very well cooked</u> and contains intestinal worms*

- *because you drink <u>dirty water</u>.*

IF YOU WANT TO PROTECT THE PEOPLE IN YOUR VILLAGE

AGAINST INTESTINAL WORMS, TELL THEM AND SHOW THEM

HOW:

- *TO BUILD AND USE <u>CLEAN LATRINES</u>*

- *TO EAT IN A CLEAN WAY (CLEAN HANDS, CLEAN FOOD,*

    WELL-COOKED MEAT)

- *TO DRINK IN A CLEAN WAY.*

WHEN A PATIENT COMES TO SEE YOU BECAUSE OF INTESTINAL WORMS,

REMIND HIM OF THE ADVICE GIVEN ABOVE AND carry out THE FOLLOWING

INSTRUCTIONS FOR TREATMENT:

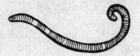

roundworm

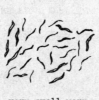

very small worm

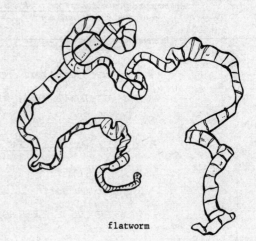

flatworm

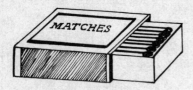

the matchbox
helps to compare
their size

a few rings of the
flatworm which fall
into the underclothes

INTESTINAL WORMS

Intestinal worms can be seen in the stools. When a patient tells
you he has worms in his stools, these worms may be round like a pencil,
or white like a ribbon, or very small like a thread.

1. IF IT IS ROUND LIKE A PENCIL

    1.1 If the patient is a child under six years old

        1.1.1 The child has no complaints or sometimes has a little
                 pain in the belly.
               Give this child some piperazine (see technique, page 251)
               Ask the parents if there are others in the family who have
                 worms and, if so, treat them also.

               Do not forget to advise the family:

               (a) to use clean latrines
               (b) to wash their hands well before they eat and
                      after they defecate
               (c) to drink clean water
               (d) not to eat food which has fallen on the ground
                      until it has been washed with clean water.

        1.1.2 The child often vomits and has bad pains in the belly
               Send him to the hospital or health centre
               If other children have worms, do not forget to treat
                 them also and to give the family the advice on
                 cleanliness of 1.1.1.

    1.2 If the patient is over six years old

         Give this patient some piperazine (see technique, page 251)
         Ask if there are others in the family who have worms and,
           if so, treat them.
         Do not forget to repeat the advice on cleanliness of 1.1.1.

2. IF IT IS WHITE LIKE A RIBBON

    Give the patient some mepacrine tablets (see page 250)
    Ask if there are others in the family who have worms and, if so,
      treat them.
    Do not forget to repeat the advice on cleanliness. Insist on the
      need to cook beef and pork well before eating it.

3. IF IT IS VERY SMALL LIKE A THREAD

    The skin around the anus itches every night.
    Give the patient piperazine tablets (see technique, page 251).

TO AVOID CATCHING WORMS
you should:

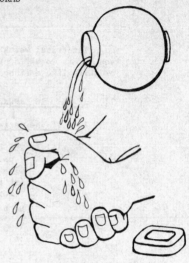

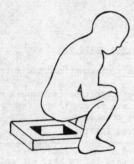

defecate in a latrine

wash your hands
before eating and after defecating

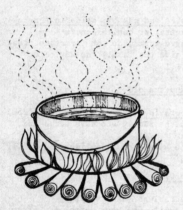

boil the water which
you are going to drink

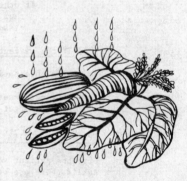

wash vegetables

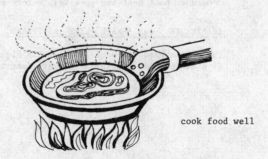

cook food well

B E   C A R E F U L :

WHEN SOMEONE HAS INTESTINAL WORMS, YOU SHOULD SEE IF OTHERS IN THE FAMILY ALSO HAVE WORMS. IF THEY DO, YOU SHOULD TREAT THEM IN THE SAME WAY.

DO NOT FORGET THAT IT IS GOOD TO TREAT PEOPLE WHO HAVE WORMS BUT EVEN BETTER TO PREVENT THEM FROM GETTING THEM.

———

WEAKNESS

AND

TIREDNESS

YOU MAY FEEL WEAK AND TIRED FOR THREE REASONS:

1. YOU ARE LOSING BLOOD

2. YOU ARE NOT EATING ENOUGH GOOD FOOD

3. SOMETHING IN THE BODY IS NOT HEALTHY.

BUT OFTEN IT IS BECAUSE YOU ARE NOT EATING ENOUGH GOOD
FOOD.

WEAKNESS AND TIREDNESS

LEARNING OBJECTIVES

At the end of his training, the PHW should be able to:

1. Talk with the people about how to keep well and prevent weakness and tiredness

2. Recognize a person who is always weak and tired

3. Recognize the signs of sudden weakness

4. Decide whether the ankles are swollen

5. Recognize when the inside of the eye is yellow, red, pink or pale (white)

6. Recognize danger signs of bleeding in pregnant women

7. Decide whether a woman is bleeding too much during her monthly period

8. Decide when someone who feels tired and weak should be sent to the hospital or health centre.

W E A K N E S S   A N D   T I R E D N E S S

1. *Either the patient has felt tired and
    weak for some time*

2. *Or the patient became weak all of a sudden*

1. THE PATIENT HAS FELT WEAK AND TIRED FOR SOME TIME

1.1 If the patient is a man or a child

  1.1.1 If there is one of the two following signs,
       send the patient to the hospital or health centre

    1. the ankles are swollen: to find out

       - press with your finger on the ankle or the
         foot for two to three seconds
       - take your finger off and see if your finger
         has left a small dent at that spot (see
         drawing No.1). If so, the ankle is swollen.

    2. the inside of the eyes is yellow: to find out

       - pull down the lower eyelid and look inside
         the eye (see drawing No.2)
         Normally the inside of the eye is pink.

  1.1.2 If there is neither of the two signs (see 1.1.1) then
       take the patient's temperature

    Either he is feverish, see Problem 1.2 "Fever"

    Or he is not feverish, but:

    1. the inside of the eyes is pale:

       - give him some iron sulfate (see technique, page 250)
       - tell the patient to rest and eat well; if possible,
         to eat meat, vegetables, eggs, fruit
       - send him to the hospital or health centre

    2. The inside of the eyes is not pale:

       - tell the patient to rest and to eat well; if possible,
         to eat meat, vegetables, eggs, fruit
       - send him to the hospital or health centre if he is not
         better after two weeks.

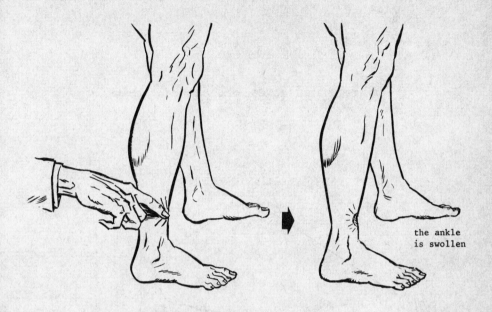

the ankle
is swollen

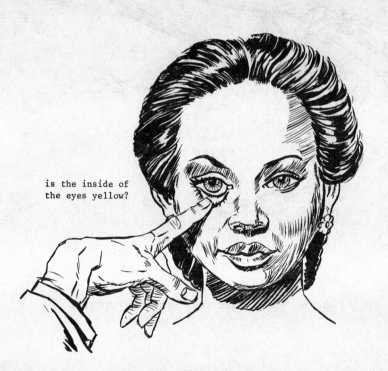

is the inside of
the eyes yellow?

DID   THE   PATIENT   BECOME   WEAK   ALL   OF   A   SUDDEN?

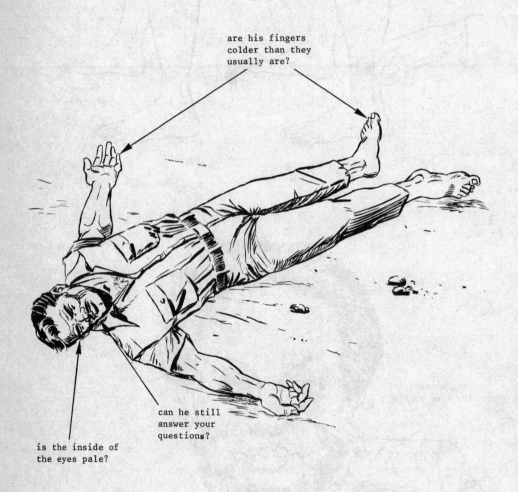

are his fingers
colder than they
usually are?

can he still
answer your
questions?

is the inside of
the eyes pale?

SEND   HIM   QUICKLY   TO   THE   HOSPITAL   OR   THE   HEALTH   CENTRE

WEAKNESS AND TIREDNESS

1.2 If the patient is a woman

1.2.1 The woman is pregnant or has just had a baby
See Problems "Pregnancy" or "After the delivery"

1.2.2 The woman is not pregnant
(a) She is losing blood through the vagina when she does not have her period, or she loses too much blood during her period.

Send her to the hospital or health centre

(b) She is not losing any blood through her vagina. Then see 1.1 as for the man and the child.

2. THE PATIENT BECAME WEAK ALL OF A SUDDEN

In that case, send him to the hospital or health centre immediately.

To find out:

2.1 Ask the patient or his family what happened: did the patient lose a lot of blood; did he feel as if he had been hit over the head?

2.2 Look for the signs of great weakness, that is:

2.2.1 The inside of the eyes is pale or yellow

2.2.2 The fingers feel colder than usual

2.2.3 The patient no longer answers your questions.

BE CAREFUL :

TO AVOID WEAKNESS AND TIREDNESS, PEOPLE SHOULD EAT GOOD FOOD:

1.   EAT FOOD WHICH CONTAINS IRON: VEGETABLES WITH GREEN LEAVES, FISH, MEAT, EGGS

2.   PREPARE FOOD IN A CLEAN WAY (See Problem 5.4)

DISEASES

OF THE MOUTH

AND TEETH

---

*TO HAVE A DISEASE OF THE MOUTH OR TEETH IS TO HAVE
EITHER A PAIN IN A TOOTH OR AROUND A TOOTH, OR TO HAVE
A PAIN WHEN YOU SWALLOW OR TO HAVE A PAIN IN THE JAW
AFTER AN ACCIDENT.*

*SINCE YOU HAVE TO EAT TO LIVE, AND SINCE TO EAT YOU
NEED TEETH WHICH CUT FOOD INTO SMALL PIECES, YOU SHOULD
TEACH THE PEOPLE TO LOOK AFTER THEIR TEETH TO STAY IN GOOD
HEALTH.*

DISEASES OF THE MOUTH AND TEETH

LEARNING OBJECTIVES

At the end of his training, the PHW should be able to:

1.   Test whether or not a patient can open his mouth

2.   Send to hospital immediately a patient who cannot open
       his mouth

3.   Find out whether a tooth hurts when it is tapped

4.   Treat a patient who is feverish and has a tooth
       that hurts when it is tapped

5.   Show a patient how to use a mouthwash and how to
       prepare salt water

6.   Treat a patient whose mouth hurts every time he
       swallows something:
           - when the patient is feverish
           - when the patient is not feverish

7.   Indicate to village people how to keep the mouth and
       teeth healthy and avoid toothache

DISEASES OF THE MOUTH AND TEETH

YOUR MOUTH AND TEETH HURT

- because you <u>do not clean</u> your mouth and teeth after you have eaten. Therefore little bits of food stay between the teeth and damage the teeth.

- because you eat <u>food which is too sugary</u>, such as sweets and cakes, and they too damage the teeth, especially when you eat them between meals

- because you <u>eat badly</u> (meals at irregular times and not enough to eat)

TO AVOID DISEASES OF THE MOUTH AND TEETH IN YOUR COMMUNITY, TELL AND SHOW THE PEOPLE HOW THEY SHOULD LOOK AFTER THEIR TEETH BY DOING THE FOLLOWING THREE THINGS :

1. CLEANING THE MOUTH AND TEETH AFTER MEALS

Either rinse the mouth with a little water after meals
or brush the teeth after meals with a toothbrush dipped in water

2. NOT TO GIVE CHILDREN TOO MANY SWEETS AND CAKES, ESPECIALLY BETWEEN MEALS

3. TO EAT FOOD WHICH PROTECTS THE HEALTH OF THE TEETH

For example, fresh fruit and vegetables, coconut, taro, sweet potato.

WHEN YOU SEE A CASE OF DISEASE OF THE MOUTH OR TEETH, REPEAT THE ADVICE GIVEN ABOVE TO THE PATIENT AND HIS FAMILY

and carry out the FOLLOWING INSTRUCTIONS FOR TREATMENT:

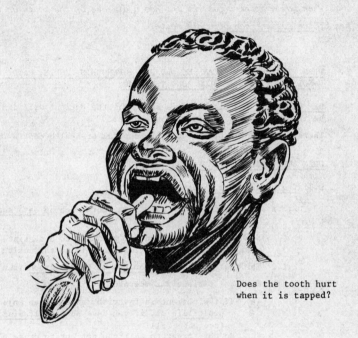

Does the tooth hurt
when it is tapped?

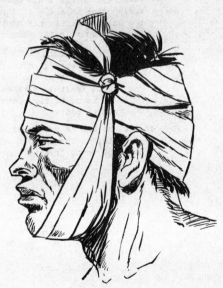

bandage to secure
the jaw

When you examine a patient who has a disease of the mouth or teeth,
see if the patient can open his mouth.

1. **WHEN THE PATIENT CAN NO LONGER OPEN HIS MOUTH, AND HAS NOT RECEIVED A BLOW ON THE JAW**

   BE CAREFUL: The situation is serious: the patient will die if he is not treated immediately by a doctor.

   Therefore send the patient to the hospital or health centre immediately.

2. **WHEN THE PATIENT CAN OPEN HIS MOUTH**

   2.1 The patient has a pain in a tooth

   2.1.1 The patient has a pain in a tooth when he eats something hot or cold

   Send this patient whenever possible to a dentist, who will treat the tooth, or send him to the health centre.

   2.1.2 The tooth hurts when you tap it with a spoon (see drawing)

   Take the patient's temperature.

   (a) If the patient is feverish, give him an injection of penicillin or, if you have none, sulfadiazine tablets (see page 251)
   Do not forget to tell the patient to drink plenty of water and to rinse his mouth with salty water (one teaspoonful in a cup of warm water). He should keep the salty water in his mouth for two to three minutes and then spit it out (and not swallow the salty water)

   See the patient again after three days:
   - if he is better, advise him to go, if possible, to the dentist or the health centre to have the tooth treated or taken out
   - if he is no better, send him to the hospital or health centre.

   (b) If the patient is not feverish, advise him to go, if possible, to the dentist or the health centre to have the tooth treated or taken out.

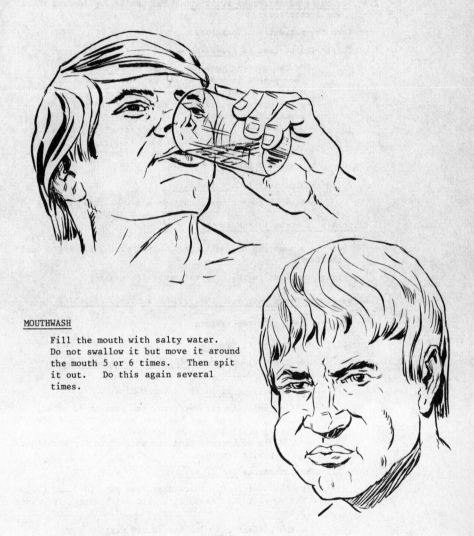

MOUTHWASH

Fill the mouth with salty water.
Do not swallow it but move it around
the mouth 5 or 6 times.   Then spit
it out.   Do this again several
times.

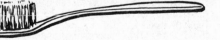

toothbrush, for cleaning teeth

2.2 <u>Something hurts around the teeth</u>. The gum is swollen and there
are little sores

Take the patient's temperature

2.2.1 The patient is <u>feverish</u>

Give the patient some <u>penicillin</u> or <u>sulfadiazine</u>
(see page 251) and tell the patient to rinse his
mouth with salty water (see 2.1.2 (a))

See the patient again after three days and tap each
tooth with a spoon

- if no tooth hurts, advise the patient to do the
  three things advised on page 200.
- if there is a tooth which hurts when you tap it
  with a spoon, see 2.1.2.

2.2.2 The patient is <u>not feverish</u>

Mouthwash four times a day for one week (see drawing)

2.3 <u>Something hurts in the mouth</u>

There is a swelling or small sores in the mouth, but not around
the teeth.

Send the patient to the hospital or health centre.

2.4 <u>Something hurts only when the patient swallows something</u>

Take the patient's temperature.

2.4.1 The patient is <u>feverish</u>

Give the patient some <u>penicillin</u> or <u>sulfadiazine</u>
(see page 251)

<u>See</u> the patient <u>again</u> after three days:

- if he is no longer feverish, the patient is cured,
  but ask him to come back and see you if he feels
  tired or if he has swollen feet
- if he is no better, send the patient to the hospital
  or health centre.

2.4.2 The patient is <u>not feverish</u>

Give him <u>aspirin</u> for three days (see page 249) and tell
him to rinse his mouth with warm salty water four times
a day

<u>See</u> the patient <u>again</u> on the fourth day:

- if nothing hurts: he is cured
- if he is no better: send him to the hospital or
  health centre.

2.5 <u>The patient has received a heavy blow on the jaw and it hurts
a lot when he tries to open his mouth</u>

Put on a bandage to secure the jaw (see drawing) and send the
patient to the hospital or health centre.

LUMPS*

UNDER THE

SKIN

ONE OR SEVERAL LUMPS MAY APPEAR IN ANY PART OF THE BODY.

THE MOST DANGEROUS ARE THOSE YOU CAN FEEL :

- AROUND THE NECK
- IN THE CREASE OF THE SHOULDER
- IN THE CREASE OF THE THIGH

AND ESPECIALLY

IF THE PATIENT HAS LOST WEIGHT AND FEELS TIRED.

---

* Small lump or small swelling that may or may not be hard and that you can feel under the skin

LUMPS UNDER THE SKIN

LEARNING OBJECTIVES

At the end of his training, the PHW should be able to:

1. Name three places of the body where lumps under the
    skin are most dangerous

2. Explain to village people how to prevent getting
    swellings and lumps on the skin

3. Examine the lump or lumps, and find out:
    - how long the lump or lumps have been there
    - whether or not the patient is feverish
    - whether or not the lump is painful
    - whether or not the lump or lumps appeared
      after an accident

4. Show the patient how to make and put on hot compresses

5. Treat a patient who is feverish and has one or more
    lumps under his skin

6. List four signs which show that the patient must be
    sent to hospital

SOME LUMPS MAY APPEAR UNDER THE SKIN

- *because you do not wash your whole body regularly with soap and water to get rid of dust and sweat, and the skin is dirty*

- *because you do not wash regularly the clothes that you wear*

- *because you have not properly treated a wound or a skin disease*

- *because you do not eat well*

- *because you have been bitten by a bad fly.*

TO REDUCE THESE DISEASES IN YOUR VILLAGE,

ADVISE THE PEOPLE:

- *TO KEEP THEIR BODIES CLEAN*

- *TO WEAR CLEAN CLOTHES*

- *TO COME AND SEE YOU ABOUT ANY WOUND OR ANY SKIN DISEASE*

- *TO EAT WELL.*

WHEN SOMEONE COMES TO SEE YOU BECAUSE HE HAS NOTICED THAT HE HAS ONE OR SEVERAL LUMPS UNDER THE SKIN

advise him again about cleanliness and carry out the FOLLOWING INSTRUCTIONS FOR TREATMENT:

LUMPS UNDER THE SKIN

When a patient comes to see you because he has noticed that he has one or several lumps under the skin, ask him since when he has these lumps:

1. THE LUMP HAS BEEN THERE FOR LESS THAN TWO WEEKS

    Take the patient's temperature

    1.1 The patient is feverish

    1.1.1 The lump hurts

    Give the patient some penicillin or, if you have none, give him some sulfadiazine tablets (see page 251)

    Also tell the patient to put hot compresses on the lump which hurts (see drawing, page 209) and give him some aspirin.

    See the patient again on the fourth day:

    - he is better: tell him to continue with the hot compresses until the lump goes away
    - or the lump has opened and there is pus coming out: see "Wounds"
    - or the patient is still feverish and the lump hurts a lot: send the patient to the hospital or health centre.

    1.1.2 The lump does not hurt

    Tell the patient to put hot compresses on the lump (see drawing, page 209) and give him aspirin

    See the patient again on the fourth day:

    - if the patient is no longer feverish, tell him to continue with the hot compresses until the lump goes away
    - if the patient is still feverish, send him to the hospital or health centre.

2. THE LUMP HAS BEEN THERE FOR MORE THAN TWO WEEKS

    2.1 The patient complains of nothing

    The lump has been there for several months or several years, but it does not bother the patient in his life and his work.

    This is not serious: reassure the patient, but tell him to come back if he notices something which bothers him in his life or his work.

    In that case, you should send the patient to the hospital or health centre.

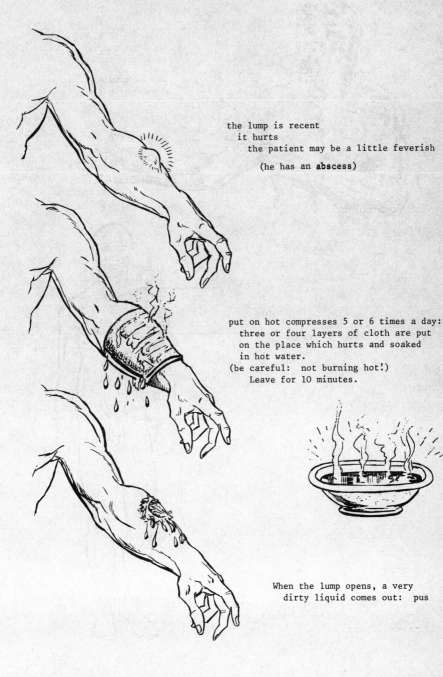

the lump is recent
  it hurts
    the patient may be a little feverish

    (he has an **abscess**)

put on hot compresses 5 or 6 times a day:
three or four layers of cloth are put
on the place which hurts and soaked
in hot water.
(be careful: not burning hot!)
Leave for 10 minutes.

When the lump opens, a very
  dirty liquid comes out: pus

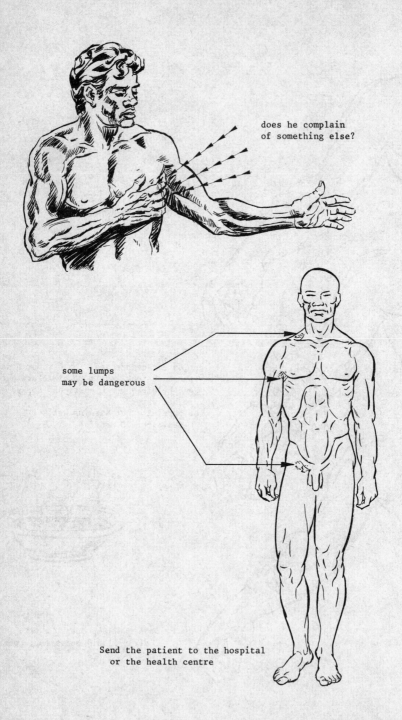

does he complain
of something else?

some lumps
may be dangerous

Send the patient to the hospital
or the health centre

2.2 The patient complains of something else

Sometimes the lump bothers the patient: he cannot see properly,
he cannot hear properly, he has difficulty in swallowing or in
breathing, he is constipated, or he cannot work or walk ...

Sometimes he feels tired, he no longer eats as he used to, he
has lost weight, he has a cough, he has diarrhoea or he is
constipated.

In all these cases, send the patient to the hospital or health
centre.

Remember that the most dangerous lumps are those you can feel:

- around the neck (in front, at the side or back)
- in the crease of the shoulder
- in the crease of the thigh (see drawing).

MENTAL

DISORDERS

TO BE IN GOOD HEALTH IS TO BE HEALTHY IN ONE'S BODY AND MIND.

ONE IS HEALTHY IN THE MIND, WHEN ONE LEARNS EASILY, IS HAPPY TO BE ALIVE, LIKES LIVING WITH OTHER PEOPLE, SOLVES ONE'S PROBLEMS AND HELPS OTHER PEOPLE TO SOLVE THEIR PROBLEMS.

MENTAL DISORDERS ARE THOSE WHICH AFFECT PEOPLE IN THEIR MINDS.

SOME PATIENTS FEEL SAD AND UNHAPPY, ARE ALWAYS TIRED, AND COMPLAIN OF PAINS IN DIFFERENT PARTS OF THEIR BODIES.

OTHERS STOP THINKING, NEVER DO ANYTHING, DO NOT MIX WITH OTHER PEOPLE ANY MORE.

OTHERS OFTEN HAVE CONVULSIONS.

SOME CHILDREN WALK AND TALK MUCH LATER THAN OTHERS OR HAVE DIFFICULTY IN LEARNING AT SCHOOL.

MENTAL DISORDERS

LEARNING OBJECTIVES

At the end of his training, the PHW should be able to:

1. Identify patients with nervous troubles, convulsions
    and other mental disorders

2. Inform people of the dangers of alcohol, wine, beer,
    coca, hashish, and of using medicines and other
    drugs too much or wrongly

3. Encourage patients to solve their own problems with
    the help of their relatives, friends, local
    authorities, etc.

4. Care for and treat patients with convulsions or
    abnormal behaviour

5. Care for children who have difficulties in learning

6. Refer to the hospital or health centre cases beyond
    his competence.

YOU CAN AND YOU MUST IMPROVE MENTAL

HEALTH IN YOUR VILLAGE/DISTRICT:

- *by looking for and helping people who complain of nervous troubles, people who have convulsions, children who have difficulty in learning and all the people who have been mentally ill for a long time*

- *by taking care of old people, especially those who forget things easily*

- *by making sure that young children are properly fed and looked after, especially those who have lost their parents or whose mothers have gone away*

- *by advising people - not to drink too much alcohol (spirits, wine or beer), especially pregnant women*
  - not to take medicines
  - not to take dangerous drugs (opium, cocaine, hashish ...)

MANY PEOPLE WHO HAVE MENTAL DISORDERS ARE TREATED AND ADVISED BY HEALERS OR PRIESTS IN THE VILLAGE OR DISTRICT. YOU SHOULD VISIT THESE HEALERS OR PRIESTS AND TALK TO THEM. TRY NOT TO OPPOSE THEM BUT, ON THE CONTRARY, OFFER YOUR HELP. THE TREATMENT THAT YOU MAY SUGGEST CAN SUPPLEMENT THEIR SKILLS. TRY TO WORK TOGETHER. ALSO TELL THEM TO CALL ON YOU IF THEY NEED HELP.[1]

----

[1] *This paragraph is typical of those which do not necessarily apply to all countries and all situations. It should be adapted to the conditions of each country.*

MENTAL DISORDERS

1. IF THE PATIENT COMPLAINS OF NERVOUS TROUBLE

The patient tells you he feels weak and gets tired easily,
                    he has pains in his head, his belly, his arms, his legs,
                    he has no appetite,
                    he has difficulty in getting to sleep or wakes very
                        early,
                    he has lost interest in sex
but above all he comes back to see you often because there is something
new wrong with him, or because he has pains in many parts of his body.

Let the patient talk and listen carefully to what he says.

Ask him if he is worried because:

- of family quarrels (with his wife, his children, his parents)
- he has no children or has too many
- he has no money
- he is having difficulties at school or at work
- he is having quarrels in the village (with his neighbours)
- he is the victim of evil spirits ...

1.1 If you think he has nervous trouble: arrange to speak to the
    patient and his closest relative. If you have no time that
    day, tell him to come back another day.

    Do not give him any medicines but tell the patient and his family
    he will get better. Try to find someone in the village who can
    help him solve his problems (a friend, the village chief, his
    boss, a clergyman, the teacher ...)

    If he does not get better, or he cannot sleep or wakes very early,
    feels sad, cries a lot, stops eating or working, send him to the
    hospital or health centre.

1.2 If you think that the patient probably does not have nervous trouble:
    find out

    - if the temperature is more than 38°C
    - or he has a cough
    - or he is pale.

    In these cases, see "Fever"
                    "Respiratory diseases" or
                    "Weakness and tiredness".

2. IF, DURING THE PREVIOUS FEW DAYS, THE PATIENT HAS BEEN FEELING
   STRANGE OR DOES NOT THINK OR BEHAVE LIKE OTHER PEOPLE

- He does not talk normally or says strange things
- Or he sees or hears things which other people do not see or hear
- Or he no longer knows where he is or what he should do
- Or he is angry or shouts or fights for no reason
- Or he no longer washes or dresses or works
- Or he runs away from home or refuses to speak or eat

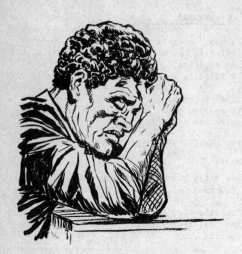

This patient is always sad

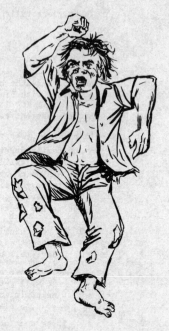

This patient behaves in a strange way

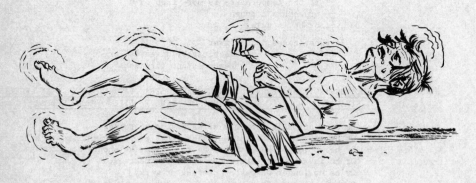

This one has convulsions

MENTAL DISORDERS

In all these cases, you should get in touch with the police, the
religious authorities and the people in the village/district and
tell everyone that this patient needs to be treated, that they must
not beat him, or shut him up somewhere, or make him leave the village,
but that they must be kind to him and put him in a quiet place. Talk
to him in a kind way and make sure that there are not too many people
around him.

Examine the patient: take his temperature.

If he has a temperature of 38°C or more: send him to the hospital or
health centre.

If he has a temperature less than 38°C:

    (a) The patient has perhaps drunk too much alcohol:
        let him sleep for a few hours and, if he is no
        better then, send him to the hospital or health
        centre.

    (b) The patient has perhaps received a blow on the head:
        send him to the hospital or health centre.

    (c) The patient has not drunk too much alcohol and has not
        received a blow on the head:
        give him chlorpromazine (see page 249), two tablets
        morning, noon and night for two days. Reassure the
        family and tell them to give the patient something
        to eat and drink, not to tie him up and to be kind
        to him.
       See the patient again after the two days' treatment.
       If he is better, continue with the chlorpromazine for
       two weeks and see him every two days.
       If he is no better, send him to the hospital or health
       centre.

3.   IF THE PATIENT HAS A CONVULSION OR CONVULSIONS

The patient falls down and no longer answers questions:

- his whole body becomes stiff
- then he has violent movements in his arms and legs
- he has foam (sometimes with blood in it) around the mouth and
  sometimes he may urinate

After some time he begins to answer when you speak to him, but he
does not remember what happened.

Always try to find someone who saw the convulsion to make sure that
it was a real convulsion, because the patient will not remember it.

If it was a real convulsion, put the patient in a quiet place and take
his temperature.

3.1 If the temperature is more than 38°C

If the patient is a child of less than two years old, give him
some aspirin (see page 249).

If the patient is a child of more than two years old, give him
some aspirin and some chloroquine (see page 249) and send him
to the hospital or health centre.

If the patient is an adult, send him to the hospital or health
centre.

3.2 If the temperature is less than 38°C

If the patient is a child under two years old, do nothing but see
him again on the following day. If the convulsions have continued,
send him to the hospital or health centre. If there have been no
more convulsions, ask the family to bring him back if the convulsions
recur.

If the patient is a child over two years old:

- Either there was only one convulsion: do nothing and see the
    child again a week later.
  If then there were no more convulsions, ask the family to bring
    the child back if the convulsions recur.
  If the child continues to have convulsions, send him to the
    hospital or health centre.

- Or there were several convulsions: give him phenobarbital for
    six months, but see him every month. For treatment with
    phenobarbital, see page 251.
  If the convulsions continue in spite of the treatment, send
    him to the hospital or health centre.

If the patient is an adult: for how long has he been having
convulsions?

- For less than a year: send him to the hospital or health
    centre.
- For more than a year: give him phenobarbital.

4. SOME CHILDREN HAVE DIFFICULTY IN LEARNING (or learn more slowly
    than the other children)

They are children who walk or talk later than the others. At school
they do not learn like the others.

You should find these children by talking with the mothers who bring
you their children when they are ill, and by talking with the village
teachers, especially those who teach first and second year schoolchildren.

Ask to see children:

who, at two years old, cannot walk on their own
who, at three years old, cannot talk properly
who cannot learn anything at school.

MENTAL DISORDERS

Then examine them:

- Is the child well fed? Weigh him and measure him, and see "The badly-fed child".

- Can the child hear properly? Talk to him very softly behind his head. If he cannot hear you, send him to the hospital or health centre.

- Can the child see properly? Show him a drawing or a book and ask him to tell you what he can see or read. If he is unable to, send him to the hospital or health centre.

- Has the child lost his parents or has his mother gone away? Try to find out who is looking after him. Is he well fed and well cared-for? If not, get in touch with the family or the village chief or the religious authorities.

- Does the child have convulsions? See paragraph (c), page 217.

- Does the child have stiffness in the arms or legs? The child cannot bend his arms and legs like other children: send him to the hospital or health centre.

But, whenever you see such children, explain clearly to their mothers and teachers how they can help them become useful and happy people. Even if they learn only slowly, they should be kept in school and later they should be trained for a job that is easy and suits their taste and ability.

5. <u>IF FOR SEVERAL MONTHS OR YEARS THE PATIENT HAS BEEN HAVING STRANGE IDEAS OR DOING STRANGE THINGS</u>

For example, the patient has been:

- Keeping to himself and talking to himself most of the time
- Getting angry when no one has done anything to him
- Frightening other people in his family or in the village
- Not working or working very little
- Not getting dressed or washing anymore.

You should look after such patients:

(1) First, you should find them. To do so, get in touch with their families, the village chief, the police, the village or district authorities.

(2) If the family has got rid of the patient and he is no better away from the family, tell them to take him back and to find him a little job in the village or district

(3) Send the patient to the hospital or health centre for treatment

(4) Visit the patient at home each month and make sure:
- he is taking his medicine regularly
- he works regularly
- the family is dealing with him properly

HOW TO IMPROVE LIFE

IN THE VILLAGE

LIFE IN THE VILLAGE HAS TO BE IMPROVED BY THE VILLAGERS THEMSELVES WITH THE HELP OF THE PHW.

THE VILLAGERS SHOULD MEET TOGETHER TO DISCUSS THE PROBLEMS OF THE VILLAGE AND DECIDE WHAT TO DO ABOUT THEM.

ALL THE PEOPLE IN THE VILLAGE CANNOT MEET AT THE SAME TIME TO TALK ABOUT VILLAGE PROBLEMS. THE PEOPLE SHOULD SELECT SEVERAL VILLAGE MEMBERS (UP TO TEN), BOTH MEN AND WOMEN, TO FORM A COMMITTEE TO TALK FOR EVERYBODY IN THE VILLAGE.

THE COMMITTEE WILL MEET REGULARLY WITH THE PHW. FOR INSTANCE, THEY CAN MEET ON THE FIRST DAY OF THE MONTH AT THE HOUSE OF THE CHIEF OR AT THE VILLAGE MEETING-PLACE.

THE COMMITTEE COULD BE CALLED THE VILLAGE HEALTH COMMITTEE IF IT TALKS ONLY ABOUT THE HEALTH OF THE VILLAGERS. IF IT TALKS ABOUT IMPROVING HEALTH AND OTHER CONDITIONS IN THE VILLAGE, IT COULD BE CALLED THE COMMUNITY DEVELOPMENT COMMITTEE, OR ANY OTHER NAME SUGGESTED BY THE LOCAL AUTHORITIES. HERE, WE SHALL CALL IT THE VILLAGE COMMITTEE.

This problem goes beyond the field of health. It is included here to prepare PHWs for their role in the development of their communities and to show how health and development problems are linked.

HOW TO IMPROVE LIFE IN THE VILLAGE

LEARNING OBJECTIVES

At the end of his training, the PHW should be able to:

1. Take an active part in village committee meetings by listening, discussing, reporting and seeking advice and help

2. Inform his supervisor about the problems of the village, report on his work, discuss his plans and obtain the supervisor's guidance and support

3. Obtain the support of the villagers in doing what the village committee and the supervisor suggest to improve life in the village

HOW TO IMPROVE LIFE IN THE VILLAGE

THE PHW HELPS TO IMPROVE LIFE IN THE VILLAGE. HE :

1. TAKES PART IN VILLAGE COMMITTEE MEETINGS

2. DISCUSSES VILLAGE PROBLEMS WITH HIS SUPERVISOR

*3. CARRIES OUT THE INSTRUCTIONS OF THE VILLAGE
   COMMITTEE AND OF HIS SUPERVISOR TO IMPROVE
   LIFE AND HEALTH IN THE VILLAGE*

1. **THE PHW TAKES PART IN VILLAGE COMMITTEE MEETINGS**

   1.1 <u>Listen</u> to what the village chief and the people say about
       village problems

   1.2 In order to have a useful discussion, <u>ask the chief</u> to help
       every member of the committee to talk about the important
       village problems

   1.3 <u>Try to answer questions</u> that the chief or people ask about
       improving village life

   1.4 <u>Talk about village health problems</u> at each meeting. <u>Say</u>
       what has been done, what has not been done and why, and
       what else could be done to improve health

   1.5 <u>Ask the committee</u> what you should do before its next
       meeting

   1.6 <u>Ask the chief</u> when the committee will next meet

   1.7 <u>Ask the people</u> to help you in your work

2. **THE PHW DISCUSSES VILLAGE PROBLEMS WITH HIS SUPERVISOR
   TO GET HIS ADVICE**

   2.1 <u>Say</u> what the problems are, what the village committee thinks
       and what it has told you to do about the problems

   2.2 <u>Tell your supervisor</u> what has been done about these problems,
       what has not been done, and why things could not be done

   2.3 <u>Ask the advice</u> of your supervisor

   2.4 <u>Bring your supervisor</u> from time to time to discuss important
       problems with the chief and the village authorities

   2.5 <u>Ask the village chief</u> to invite your supervisor to village
       committee meetings from time to time to talk with the
       members

   2.6 <u>Tell your supervisor</u> regularly what you need for your work
       in the village (medicines, supplies ...)

3. THE PHW CARRIES OUT THE INSTRUCTIONS OF THE VILLAGE
    COMMITTEE AND HIS SUPERVISOR TO IMPROVE LIFE IN
    THE VILLAGE

    3.1 Work with the villagers to clean the village and the houses
         and to keep them clean:

         - Organize cleaning teams (sweepers, pavers ...)
         - Promote use of concrete or tile floors in houses
         - Make roofs more watertight
         - Improve sanitation (see "Excreta disposal", page 136;
           "Waste disposal", page 142; "Food protection", page 149)
         - Build fences and shelters for animals to keep them out of
           the houses
         - Dig drainage ditches to remove water from the streets and
           courtyards after rain

    3.2 Work with the villagers to improve other village conditions,
         such as:

         - Water supply for drinking and irrigation of crops
           (see "Water supply", page 129)
         - Water storage (tanks, reservoirs, cisterns ...)
         - Education of children and adults
         - Recreation areas for children and adults
         - Electricity for homes and work
         - Roads and paths for better access to the village
         - Communication with outside villages (see "Improving transport
           and communication", page 232)

    3.3 Work to increase production and employment in the village:

              What new foods can be grown in the village?
              What can be done to increase animal breeding?
              What kind of local industry and handicrafts can be
                developed or improved?
              What kind of services could visit the village
                regularly (library, bus, bank, merchants, postal
                service ...)?

    3.4 Visit people in their homes to see what their main needs are
         and how to meet these needs.

FOODSTUFFS*

TO STAY IN GOOD HEALTH, ONE MUST EAT. TO EAT WELL, ONE MUST OBEY TWO RULES :

1. EAT ENOUGH (OTHERWISE PEOPLE WILL NOT HAVE THE STRENGTH TO WORK)

2. EAT VARIED FOODS (OTHERWISE PEOPLE WILL CATCH DISEASES).

YOU SHOULD TAKE AN INTEREST IN WHAT THE PEOPLE IN YOUR VILLAGE OR DISTRICT EAT. YOU SHOULD TRY TO IMPROVE THEIR DIET.

---

*This problem also goes beyond the field of health. It is included here to prepare PHWs for their role in the development of their communities and to show how health and development problems are linked.

FOODSTUFFS

LEARNING OBJECTIVES

At the end of his training, the PHW should be able to:

1. Identify foods that local people do not like to eat

2. Tell the people which are the best local foods to eat

3. Explain to farmers, the village chief and community development workers how to grow new foods

4. Organize meetings with village women to show how to prepare and cook good local food for the family

5. Give three examples of advice the PHW can give to encourage village people to grow food

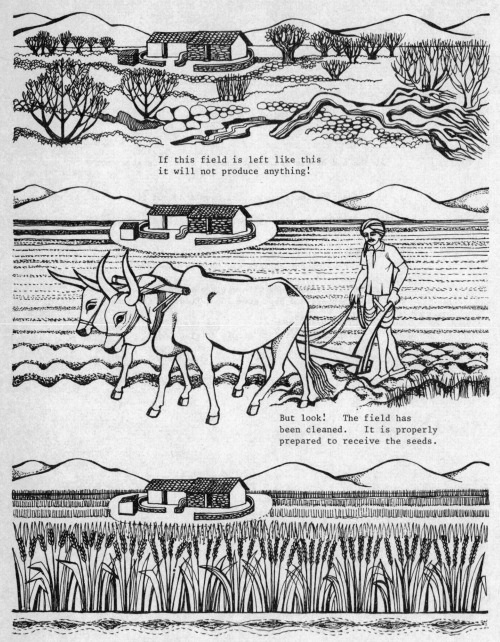

If this field is left like this
it will not produce anything!

But look! The field has
been cleaned. It is properly
prepared to receive the seeds.

The field has been sown.
The wheat or the rice has grown.
Now the village will be able
to eat more.

*Some children are not growing as quickly as others <u>or</u> the people
in the village complain that there is no food <u>or</u> your supervisor asks
you what you have done to improve the diet of the children, the men
and the women.*

WHAT WILL YOU DO ?

1. FIND OUT IF THERE ARE SOME FOODS WHICH THE PEOPLE
   DO NOT LIKE TO EAT

2. FIND OUT IF THEY CAN PRODUCE NEW FOODS IN THE
   VILLAGE

3. ORGANIZE A MEETING WITH THE VILLAGE COMMITTEE

1. <u>ARE THERE SOME FOODS WHICH THE PEOPLE IN THE VILLAGE
   DO NOT LIKE TO EAT?</u>

   1.1 <u>YES</u> People have always said that some foods were not good
        or that it was forbidden to touch them

        1.1.1 <u>Make a list</u> of these foods

        1.1.2 <u>Tell the village chief</u> which foods the people should
              eat, foods which your supervisor has advised (see 3)

   1.2 <u>NO</u> Then:

2. IS IT POSSIBLE TO PRODUCE NEW FOODS IN THE VILLAGE?

   2.1 <u>YES</u>

       2.1.1 Is there unused land that can be farmed?

       2.1.2 Are there new seeds that can be bought?

       2.1.3 Is there water for the land and for the cattle?

       2.1.4 Can fertilizer be made by leaving plant waste (leaves,
             vegetables, roots, fruit) in a hole for about two
             months?

       2.1.5 Can more cattle be reared?

   If so, <u>tell the village chief</u> that the people suffer from eating too
   little and that this will change if more food is produced in the
   village. <u>Ask the chief</u> to arrange a meeting with the important
   people in the village.

A GOOD HARVEST
MUST BE PREPARED!

TO HAVE THIS

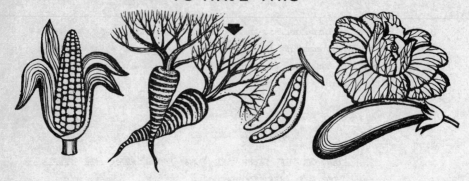

DO THIS

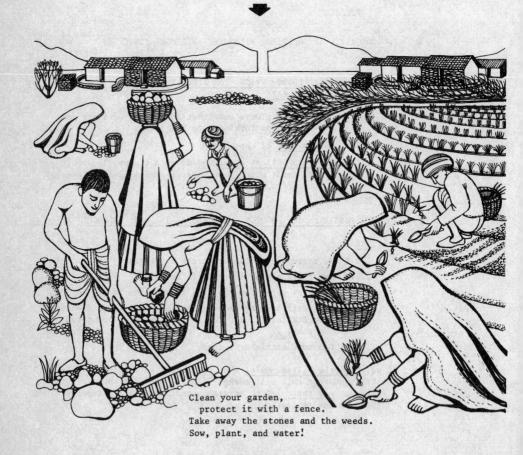

Clean your garden,
  protect it with a fence.
Take away the stones and the weeds.
Sow, plant, and water!

FOODSTUFFS

2.2 <u>NO</u>   <u>Tell the village chief</u> that:

   2.2.1 In spite of all the food in the village, there are
       people who are ill with hunger (children, sick people,
       disabled people, unemployed people, orphans, widows ...)

   2.2.2 Something should be done: discussion with the chiefs of
       neighbouring villages, with the government, etc ...

3. <u>ORGANIZE A MEETING WITH THE VILLAGE COMMITTEE</u>

3.1 <u>Ask</u> your supervisor's opinion on points 1.2 and 2.1.

3.2 <u>Invite your supervisor</u> to the meeting with the village committee
    and <u>ask</u> him to suggest how farming and cattle-rearing might be
    improved.

3.3 <u>Listen</u> to what the supervisor says so that you can <u>repeat it</u> and
    <u>make sure</u> that his advice is followed:

   3.3.1 To improve farming. For example:

     - Fruit: to plant trees on a well-exposed piece of
       land, near the school so that the pupils can water
       them
     - Vegetables: to sow or plant in well-irrigated land ...
     - Cereals: to till large areas ...
     - Fodder: to sow seed in fields after the harvest ...

   3.3.2 To improve the rearing of animals. For example:

     - Sheep and pigs: to find foodstuffs, to watch the
       flocks ...
     - Poultry: to build a poultry yard, to watch over
       breeding.

3.4 <u>Suggest to the village committee that it discusses</u> each of your
    supervisor's suggestions for farming or cattle-rearing, in his
    presence

3.5 <u>Let it choose one or more projects</u> for farming or cattle-rearing
    (for example: growing spinach)

   <u>Tell the village committee</u> what the people must do for this project.
   For example, to grow spinach, carrots or maize, they must:

    - choose some land and prepare it; take away the stones,
      till it, cover it with animal or vegetable fertilizer
    - find seed and sow it at intervals
    - find water to water it regularly
    - build a fence to prevent the animals from destroying
      the crop

   <u>Say</u> that your supervisor can help them in this work.

3.6 <u>Ask the village committee</u> to choose a man from the village to
    supervise the new farming and cattle-rearing activities, who
    will stay in contact with you and your supervisor.

TO REAR ANIMALS
ONE MUST LOOK AFTER THEM!

Feed them
Give them something to drink
Give them shelter

TO HAVE THIS

DO THIS

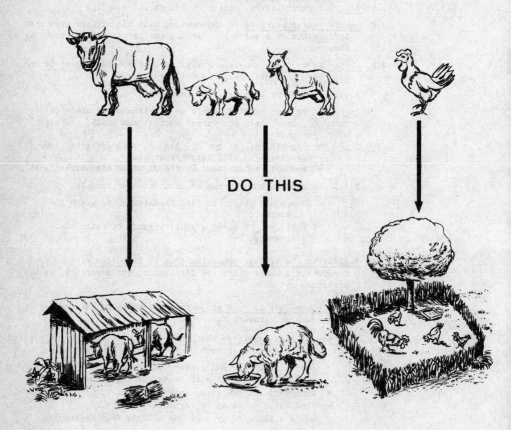

FOODSTUFFS

BE CAREFUL:

YOU WILL NOT FIND FOOD WITHOUT DOING ANYTHING ABOUT IT.

PLANTS WILL GROW ONLY IF THE FIELDS ARE PREPARED.

ANIMALS WILL GROW AND BREED ONLY IF THEY ARE GIVEN
FOOD AND WATER.

TO PRODUCE PLANTS AND REAR ANIMALS, WORK WITH OTHER PEOPLE
IN THE VILLAGE AND HELP THEM.

ABOVE ALL YOU SHOULD _RELY ON YOURSELF_ AND ON THE RESOURCES
OF THE VILLAGE TO DEVELOP THE VILLAGE AND TO IMPROVE THE LIFE
OF THE PEOPLE. _THERE IS ALWAYS SOMETHING WHICH CAN BE DONE ON
THE SPOT WITH THE MEANS OF THE VILLAGE_: YOU SHOULD LOOK FOR
POSSIBILITIES, FIND THEM, DISCUSS THEM AND THEN _ACT_.

IMPROVING TRANSPORT AND COMMUNICATION*

LEARNING OBJECTIVES

At the end of his training, the PHW should be able to:

1. Recommend a means of transport to enable the villagers
    to get to town: mule, donkey, horse, cart or bus

2. Make a stretcher

3. Explain the advantages of being able to get to town
    in a cart pulled by a donkey, a mule or a horse

4. Explain that, to get to town quickly, three things
    are needed:
    - (a) a means of transport
    - (b) someone responsible for the transport
           (driver)
    - (c) good paths

5. Ask a health worker in the next village for advice
    and show him what has been done

6. Ask important people from the town to come to the
    village to show them what has been done in the
    village and to ask their advice

---

* *This problem also goes beyond the field of health. It is included*
to prepare PHWs for their role in the development of their communities
and to show how much the problems of health and development are linked.

HOW TO BUILD A STRETCHER

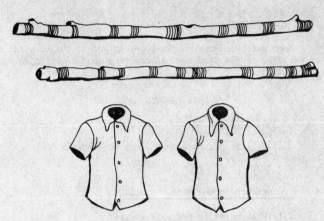

With two sticks 2 metres long
and
two shirts

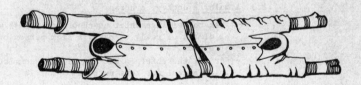

STRETCHER

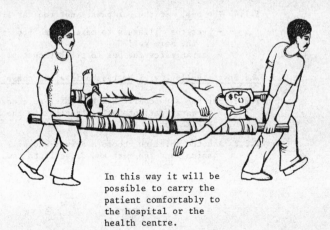

In this way it will be
possible to carry the
patient comfortably to
the hospital or the
health centre.

*Some patients have no transport to get to the hospital or health centre,
or very few people from the neighbouring town or villages ever come to visit
your village.*

WHAT   SHOULD   YOU   DO?

1.   *To get to town more quickly*

2.   *To get to your village more easily*

1.   TO   GET   TO   TOWN   MORE   QUICKLY

   1.1   Who means do you want to use?

      1.1.1   The stretcher for carrying sick people. To make a stretcher:

         - cut two strong sticks 2 metres long
         - push the sticks through two shirts, or fasten creepers
           between the sticks (see drawing)

      1.1.2   A mule, a donkey, a horse:

         - ask the village chief to choose an animal which will
           always be ready to carry a sick person or to pull
           a cart
         - or ask the chief to get the village committee to buy
           an animal for this purpose

      1.1.3   A cart:

         - ask the village committee to find a person who can
           make a cart
         - and to find an animal to pull the cart (see 1.1.2)

      1.1.4   The bus: if the bus passes not too far from the village:

         - get the villagers to make a path from the village to
           the main road
         - arrange for the bus to stop at that place

   1.2   Who in the village will be responsible for these things?

      1.2.1   For the stretcher: ask the chief to choose three people
              to carry patients on a stretcher to the hospital or
              health centre

      1.2.2   Ask the chief to choose a driver who will look after the
              animal and the cart and drive it to town

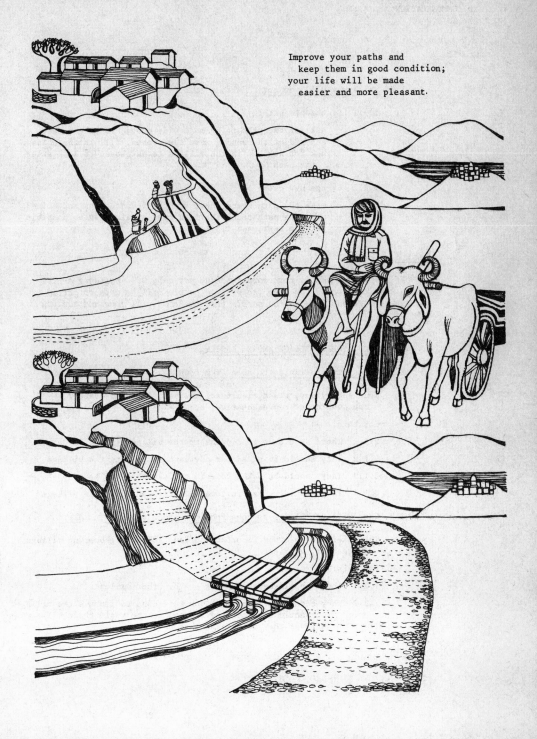

Improve your paths and
keep them in good condition;
your life will be made
easier and more pleasant.

IMPROVING TRANSPORT
AND COMMUNICATION

1.3 Which way will you go?

1.3.1 By the old path:

- ask for the path to be made wide enough to take a cart
- get rid of the weeds, move the stones, fill in the holes
- ask for someone in the village to be chosen to look after
   the path

1.3.2 By the new path:

- make the path where there are the fewest bumps and holes
- make the path reach the main road as directly as possible
- for the rest, see 1.3.1

N O T E :

If people can get to town more quickly, not only will patients arrive at the hospital sooner but also the village people will be able to get to the market more easily, and the people from the town will come and see you more often.

2. TO REACH YOUR VILLAGE MORE EASILY

2.1 Whom will you invite to come from town?

Your supervisor, the agricultural adviser, the head teacher,
  the government representative, etc.

For this:

2.1.1 There should be good paths to the village (see 1.3)

2.1.2 They should be asked for advice on improving the village

2.1.3 They should be asked to come and see what you have done

2.1.4 They should be met in town and accompanied to the village

2.2 Whom will you invite to come from the other villages?

The chief or any other important person from a neighbouring village
  (a teacher, a priest ...)

For this:

2.2.1 There should be good paths to the other villages

2.2.2 They should be shown what you have done to improve the village;
       you should ask their advice and ask to visit their village
       whenever they do something good

IMPROVING TRANSPORT
AND COMMUNICATION

_N O T E_ :

THE EASIER IT IS TO USE THE TRACKS OR THE PATHS THE
EASIER IT WILL BE TO GET TO TOWN AND TO YOUR VILLAGE.

BUT GOOD TRACKS AND GOOD PATHS NEED SOME EFFORT.

THEY MUST FIRST BE MADE; THEN THEY SHOULD BE KEPT IN
GOOD CONDITION AND REPAIRED WHENEVER THEY ARE DAMAGED.

HOW TO KEEP

RECORDS

RECORDS ARE WRITTEN INFORMATION IN NOTEBOOKS ABOUT THE HEALTH OF THE PEOPLE AND THE HEALTH CONDITIONS OF THE VILLAGE.

EACH DAY THE PHW WILL WRITE IN NOTEBOOKS WHAT HE HAS DONE OR OBSERVED ABOUT THE HEALTH OF THE COMMUNITY.

RECORD NOTEBOOKS ARE ALWAYS KEPT IN A SAFE PLACE AT THE HEALTH POST.

THE INFORMATION IN THE RECORDS WILL BE USED TO :

- KNOW THE HEALTH CONDITIONS OF THE VILLAGE, INCLUDING BIRTHS AND DEATHS;

- KNOW THE STATE OF HEALTH OF THE PEOPLE AND WHAT HAS BEEN DONE TO IMPROVE IT;

- HELP TO PLAN FUTURE ACTIVITIES ON THE BASIS OF THE HEALTH NEEDS OF THE COMMUNITY.

THE RECORDS WILL BE SHOWN TO THE VILLAGE COMMITTEE AND TO THE SUPERVISOR. THE PHW, WITH THE AGREEMENT AND SUPPORT OF THE VILLAGE COMMITTEE AND HIS SUPERVISOR, WILL USE HIS RECORDS AS A BASIS FOR DECISIONS AND ACTIONS.

HOW TO KEEP RECORDS

The PHW will record each day in his notebook(s):

1.   The births and deaths which have occurred in the village;

2.   The people he has seen in the health post and what action
     he has taken;

3.   The people he has seen in their homes and what action he
     has taken;

4.   All his other activities to improve the health conditions
     of the village.

How this information will be recorded will differ from country to
country. The following format is given only as an example. It should be
ADAPTED to the requirements of each health service. An attempt has been
made to keep the example as simple as possible.

1.   Births will be recorded with the following information:

               - date of birth
               - name of child
               - sex of child
               - names and place of residence of parents
               - name of person assisting with birth
               - whether the child was born alive or dead

This information could be written in columns in a notebook as follows:

Date of birth	Name of child	Sex		Names and place of residence of parents	Name of person assisting with birth	Child born alive?	
		M	F			Yes	No

2.   Deaths will be recorded with the following information:

               - date of death
               - name of dead person
               - sex of dead person
               - age of dead person
               - suspected cause of death
               - name of person reporting death

This information could be written in columns in the notebook, as follows:

Date of death	Name of dead person	Sex M	F	Age	Suspected cause of death	Name of person reporting death

3. The health activities of the PHW at the health post or in the homes of villagers will also be recorded in a notebook. The following information will be included:

- name of each patient seen
- age of patient
- sex of patient
- what patient complained of
- what the PHW did

This information could be written in columns in the notebook as follows:

Date	Name and place of residence of patient	Age	Sex M	F	Patient's complaint	PHW finding	Action taken

4. Other activities of the PHW will be recorded. Here the PHW will write what he has done, such as:

4.1 Prevention

Health education and advice: _____
_____

Action to improve sanitation and cleanliness in the homes and village: _____
_____

4.2 <u>Other community development activities</u>

Private meetings with local authorities: _____

_____

_____

Meetings of village committee: _____

_____

_____

Others: _____

_____

_____

IF SEVERAL NOTEBOOKS ARE NOT AVAILABLE, ONE NOTEBOOK CAN BE
DIVIDED INTO SECTIONS TO RECORD THE DIFFERENT TYPES OF
INFORMATION REQUIRED.

HOW TO MAKE REPORTS

REPORTS ARE INFORMATION WRITTEN EACH MONTH BY THE PHW TO SHOW THE MAIN THINGS HE HAS OBSERVED AND WHAT HE HAS DONE ABOUT THE HEALTH OF THE COMMUNITY DURING THE MONTH.   THE NAMES OF HIS PATIENTS SHOULD NOT BE GIVEN IN HIS REPORTS.

ON THE LAST DAY OF EACH MONTH THE PHW USES HIS RECORDS TO PREPARE HIS MONTHLY REPORT.   THIS REPORT WILL BE DISCUSSED WITH THE VILLAGE COMMITTEE AND WITH HIS SUPERVISOR.   IT WILL BE KEPT BY THE PHW IN A SAFE PLACE AT THE HEALTH POST.

THE TYPE OF REPORT, THE INFORMATION IT CONTAINS, ITS FREQUENCY AND ITS UTILIZATION WILL DIFFER FROM COUNTRY TO COUNTRY.   THE FOLLOWING FORMATS ARE GIVEN ONLY AS EXAMPLES. THEY SHOULD BE ADAPTED TO THE REQUIREMENTS OF EACH HEALTH SERVICE.   AN ATTEMPT HAS BEEN MADE TO KEEP THESE EXAMPLES AS SIMPLE AS POSSIBLE.

HOW TO MAKE REPORTS

The PHW will complete each month:

1. A health report, and

2. A medicine and supply report

1. The health report should contain the following information:

- the number of births
- the number of deaths
- the type and number of complaints
- other PHW health activities
- comments by the PHW
- comments by the village committee

This information could be written in a form such as:

HOW TO MAKE REPORTS

HEALTH REPORT FOR THE VILLAGE OF _____

YEAR _____ MONTH _____ NAME OF PHW _____

---

1.   Number of births during the month: _____ male
                                           _____ female
                                           _____ born dead

                                           _____ TOTAL BIRTHS

2.   Number of deaths during the month: _____ under 5 years old
                                           _____ over 5 years old

                                           _____ TOTAL DEATHS

3.   Number of patients seen during the month:

                                           _____ under 5 years old
                                           _____ 5 years and over

                                           _____ TOTAL PATIENTS SEEN

4.   Number of patients referred: _____.

5.   Type and number of complaints during the month:

        _____ fever   _____ burns

        _____ diarrhoea   _____ malnutrition

        _____ wounds   _____ others

     (This list will be developed as appropriate by the health services).

6.   Other PHW health activities: _____
     _____

7.   PHW comments: _____
     _____

                        * * * * * * * * *

Village Committee comments: _____

Supervisor comments: _____

---

*SOME HEALTH SERVICES MAY FIND IT CONVENIENT TO HAVE THEIR
REPORTING FORMS PRINTED AND DISTRIBUTED IN ADVANCE TO THE
PHW IN ORDER TO STANDARDIZE INFORMATION. IT COULD BE HELPFUL
TO HAVE THE FORMS PRINTED IN THREE DIFFERENT COLOURS: ONE
COLOUR FOR KEEPING AT THE HEALTH POST, ONE COLOUR FOR THE
VILLAGE COMMITTEE, AND ONE COLOUR FOR THE SUPERVISOR. IN
THAT CASE, THE PHW MUST PREPARE HIS REPORT IN TRIPLICATE.*

2. The medicine and supply report should contain the following
    information:

    - the name of the item
    - the amount remaining from the previous month
    - the amount received during the month being reported on
    - the amount used during the month being reported on
    - the amount needed for the next supply

This information could be written in a form such as:

MEDICINE AND SUPPLY REPORT FOR THE VILLAGE OF _____

YEAR _____ MONTH _____ NAME OF PHW _____

ITEM A	Remaining from previous month B	Received during the month C	Amount used during month D	Remaining at the end of the month E *	Amount requested for next supply F
(A standardized list of medicines and supplies can be used if desired. Also other items such as soap, bricks, bags of cement, etc.) 1. ... 2. ... 3. ...				* (E=B+C-D)	

The number written in Column B should be the same as the number written in
Column E of the previous month's report.

HOW TO MAKE REPORTS

3. The PHW will discuss his health report and his medicine and supply
    report at the village committee meeting. The committee can then
    see the needs and problems of the village. Members of the village
    committee can:

    - see what the PHW does
    - see how they can help him in his work
    - comment on the report
    - decide on any action which should be taken in the village

4. The PHW will discuss his reports with his supervisor. His
    supervisor will then know the state of health of the community
    and what the PHW and the village committee are doing. The
    supervisor will:

    - guide the PHW on his work and his referrals
    - advise what other actions need to be taken
    - see what supplies and medicines are needed
    - discuss the plans of the PHW for his next period of work.

ANNEXES

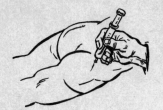

MEDICINES

How to give them
How much to give

————

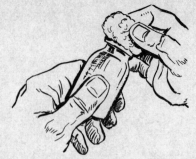

1. <u>Some general information</u>

Remember that:

1) The dosage of medicines is different for a baby under one year old, a small child (1 to 3 years old), a child (4 to 12 years old) and an adult (or a child over 12).

2) Medicines may be given in different ways:

    - by injection
    - or in tablets
    - or in drops
    - or in liquid or ointment which you put on the skin.

3) Medicine will cure the patient only if it is given in the proper way:

    - for injections, see techniques, pages 254-258
    - for tablets: for babies and children, crush the tablets
        and mix them with milk or fruit juice or treacle or jam
    - for drops, count the drops
    - for liquids or ointments, spread them on the skin with a
        clean cloth or clean cotton wool.

4) The medicine may be given once or several times. When it is given several times a day, there should be an interval between each dose (for example: one tablet at 8.00 a.m., one at noon, one at 16h00 and one at 20h00).

5) Use the list on the following pages only as instructed in a chapter of this Guide.

6) Never buy and never use medicine which you do not know: this could be very dangerous.

<u>*Important remarks:*</u>

   1.   The names of the medicines given in this Guide are the common names. Each country should specify any changes which it may wish to make in the names.

   2.   The dosages and the packaging may vary from one country to another. They should therefore be revised to adapt them to local conditions of use.

1 tablet ⬭

1/2 tablet ◲

1/4 tablet ◺

2. <u>How to use the medicines mentioned in this Guide</u>

NAME OF MEDICINE	MAINLY FOR TREATMENT OF	HOW TO GIVE IT	HOW MUCH TO GIVE			
			BABY less than 1 year old	SMALL CHILD from 1 to 3 years	CHILD from 4 to 12 years	ADULT or CHILD over 12 years old
ASPIRIN	Fever and pains	500 mg tablets	-	½	½ . . . . 3 times a day . . .	1 to 3 . . . . .
ATROPINE	Abdominal pains	intramuscular injection	-	-	-	¼ mg repeat once if necessary
AUREOMYCIN (eye ointment)	Eye diseases	ointment	Put a little ointment in the corner of the eye two or three times a day for three to five days			
BELLADONNA tincture	Abdominal pains	drops in a glass of water	-	3 drops per year of age, but no more than 30 drops		30 drops
BENZYL BENZOATE	Skin diseases	liquid to put on the skin	First wash the skin with soap and water, leave to dry; then put the liquid on the skin with a clean cloth. Repeat once a day for three days			
CHLOROQUINE	Fever (treatment of malaria)	100 mg tablets	½	1 . . . . for three days	3	6 . . . . .
CHLORPROMAZINE	Mental disorders	25 mg tablets	-	-	1 tablet . . . . . morning, noon and night for two days (more if necessary, see page 217)	2 tablets

NAME OF MEDICINE	MAINLY FOR TREATMENT OF	HOW TO GIVE IT	HOW MUCH TO GIVE			
			BABY less than 1 year old	SMALL CHILD from 1 to 3 years	CHILD from 4 to 12 years	ADULT or CHILD over 12 years old
ERGOTAMINE	Bleeding after delivery or miscarriage	1 mg tablets	-	-	-	1 to 2; repeat once or twice if necessary
GENTIAN VIOLET or TINCTURE OF IODINE	Cleaning wounds	liquid to put on skin	First wash the skin with soap and water, leave to dry then put the liquid on the skin with a clean cloth			
IRON SULFATE	Weakness Tiredness	250 mg tablets	-	-	1 to be taken with food twice a day for one month	
MEPACRINE	Against flat worms	100 mg tablets	-	4	6	10
			Laxative the night before. Tablets to be taken all together in the morning on an empty stomach			
ORAL REHYDRATION SALTS	Diarrhoea	1 packet dissolved in 1 litre of drinking water	As much as is needed to quench thirst. Then 1 to 2 cupfuls for each watery stool passed. Adults may need several litres a day. Continue until diarrhoea stops.			
OXYTOCINE	Expulsion of placenta. To stop bleeding quickly after delivery or miscarriage	Intramuscular injection ampoules of 5 IU (international units)	-	-	-	1 Intramuscular injection of contents of a 5 IU ampoule

NAME OF MEDICINE	MAINLY FOR TREATMENT OF	HOW TO GIVE IT	HOW MUCH TO GIVE			
			BABY less than 1 year old	SMALL CHILD from 1 to 3 years	CHILD from 4 to 12 years	ADULT or CHILD over 12 years old
PROCAINE PENICILLIN (aqueous solution)	Infections	Intramuscular injection	-	250 000 units	500 000 units	1 000 000 units
			every day for three days			
PHENOBARBITAL	To treat someone who has convulsions	50 mg tablets	-	½	1	1 to 2
			two or three times a day for two days; then half the dosage for six months			
PIPERAZINE	Roundworms	500 mg tablets (crushed in a spoon)	2	3 or 4	6	8
			once			
	Very small worms		½	1		1½
			three times a day for a week			
SULFADIAZINE	Infections	500 mg tablets	½	1	2	3
			to be taken with a glass of water four times a day for three days			
TETRACYCLINE	Infections	250 mg tablets	1/5	½	1	1 to 3
			four times a day for three days			

A FEW

TECHNIQUES

1. TAKING THE TEMPERATURE

There are three common ways of taking a person's temperature - by placing a thermometer in the mouth, or under the armpit, or in the anus.

1.1 If the temperature is being taken in the mouth or under the armpit

1.1.1 See that the column of mercury inside the thermometer is below about 35°C. If it is not, shake the thermometer until the line has gone down.

1.1.2 Ask the patient to place the small part of the thermometer under his tongue and to keep his mouth closed, or under his armpit and to hold his elbow against his body.

1.1.3 Leave the thermometer in place for about two minutes.

1.1.4 Take the thermometer out and read the figure which the column of mercury inside the thermometer has reached. If the figure is above 37.5°C the patient has a fever. The higher the figure is, the greater is the fever.

1.1.5 Clean the thermometer with some cotton wool and soapy water (not hot water). Shake the thermometer so that the mercury goes down towards the small part. Put the thermometer away so that it does not fall on to the ground and break.

1.2 If the temperature is being taken in the anus (see drawings on next page)

1.2.1 See that the line of mercury is below about 35°C (see 1.1.1).

1.2.2 Ask the patient to push the small part of the thermometer into his anus. If the patient is a child or is unable to do it himself, you must insert it for him.

1.2.3 Leave the thermometer in place for about two minutes. An adult should be lying on his side; a child (especially a small child) should lie on his front and you should hold him to prevent him from rolling over.

1.2.4 Remove the thermometer and read the temperature as in 1.1.4 above.

1.2.5 Clean, shake down and put away the thermometer as in 1.1.5 above.

What temperatures do these thermometers show?

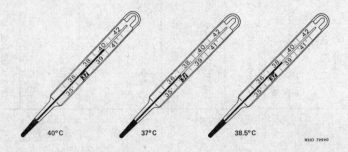

40°C   37°C   38.5°C

WHO 79990

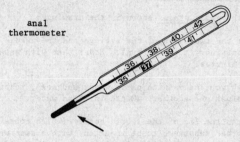

anal
thermometer

*small part
filled with mercury*

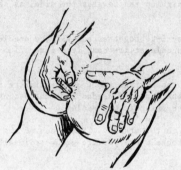

push all the small part
into the anus

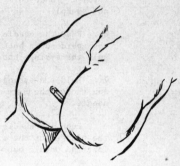

leave in for two minutes

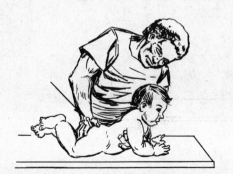

in the case of a small child
put him on a table

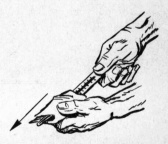

clean the thermometer

2. <u>INTRAMUSCULAR INJECTION</u> (in the buttocks)

Follow the <u>eight stages</u> shown in the drawings:

1. Put the two parts of the syringe and the needle (page 258) in a metal container (a pan or tin). Cover them with water and boil them for ten minutes.

2. Wash your hands with clean water and soap, rubbing your hands hard against one another. Rinse in clean water.

3. Clean the lid of the little bottle (which contains the penicillin or any other substance to be injected) with a swab wetted with a disinfectant such as surgical spirit, alcohol, gentian violet: rub hard two or three times.

4. With the same swab, rub the skin two or three times where you are going to insert the needle. On the buttocks choose a place for the injection which is fairly high up and towards the side, as shown in the drawing (see stage 4).

5. Put the two parts of the syringe together and fit the needle in firmly. To do this, hold the needle at its base (the part which is not sharp).

6. Push the needle fitted to the syringe about one centimetre into the upside-down bottle. Draw the quantity needed into the syringe; pull the syringe out holding the base of the needle.

7. Hold the syringe as shown in the drawing. Stand behind the patient and choose the place on the buttocks where you are going to insert the needle.

8. Push the needle in quickly about two centimetres at least. Press the plunger of the syringe until all the liquid in the syringe has gone. Take the needle out while holding <u>its base</u> still attached to the syringe.

If you have sterile disposable syringes, follow instructions 2, 3, 4, 6, 7 and 8 above.

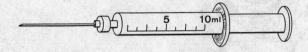

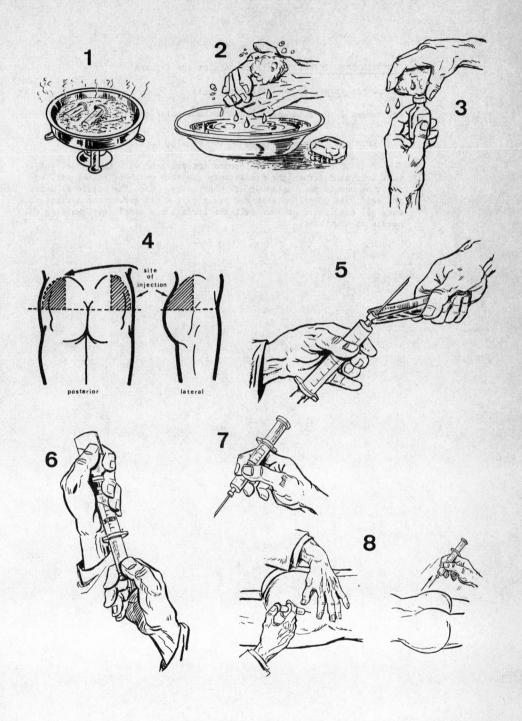

3. SUBCUTANEOUS INJECTION (in the arm or the forearm)

Follow the stages shown in the drawings:

For stages 1, 2, 3, 5 and 6, see "Intramuscular injection".

7.   Hold the syringe as shown in the drawing opposite.

8.   Pick up the skin of the forearm (or the arm) with the fingers of
your left hand. Push the needle into the skin which is pulled out, so
that the needle goes in about one centimetre. Once the needle is under
the skin, let go of the skin and press on the plunger of the syringe to
make all the liquid go in. Pull the syringe and needle out, holding the
needle at its base.

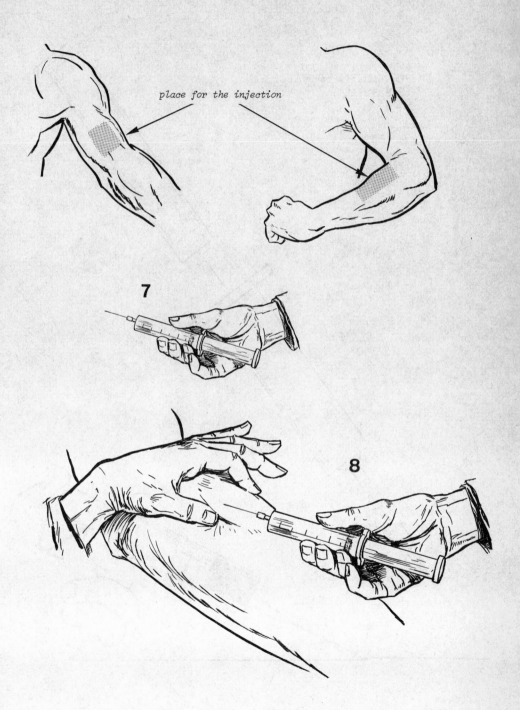

place for the injection

7

8

The different parts
of a syringe

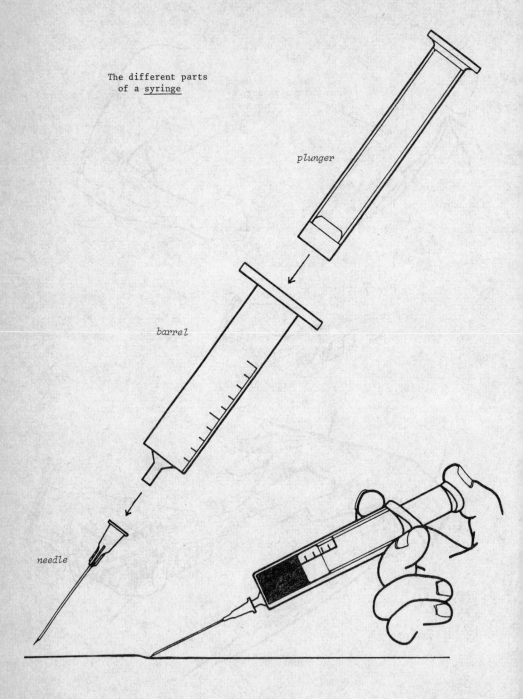

plunger

barrel

needle

4. A FEW EXAMPLES OF BANDAGES

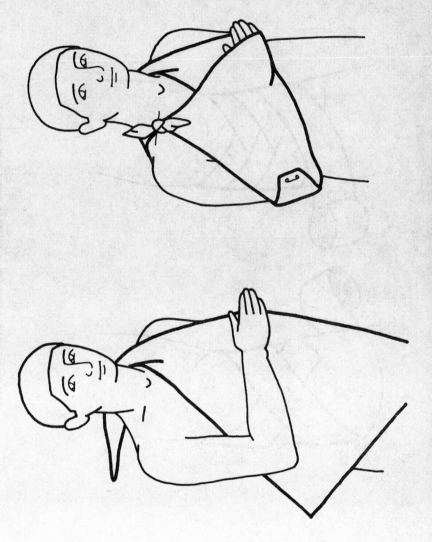

ARM SLING / BRAS EN ÉCHARPE

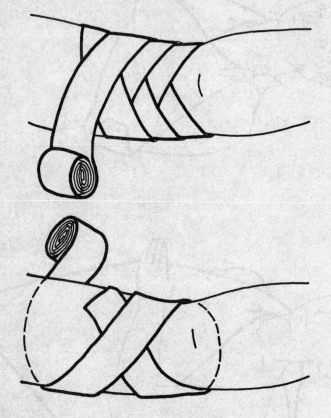

ROLLER BANDAGE : UPPER ARM / BANDAGE CIRCULAIRE - BRAS

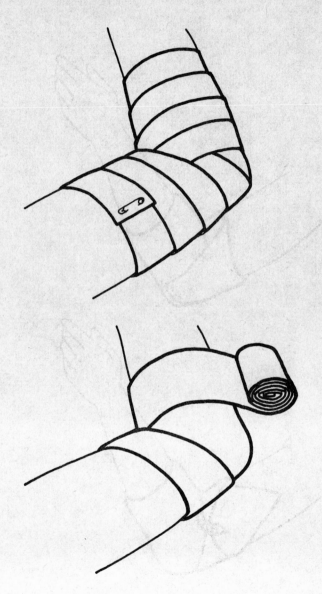

ROLLER BANDAGE: ELBOW / BANDAGE CIRCULAIRE - COUDE

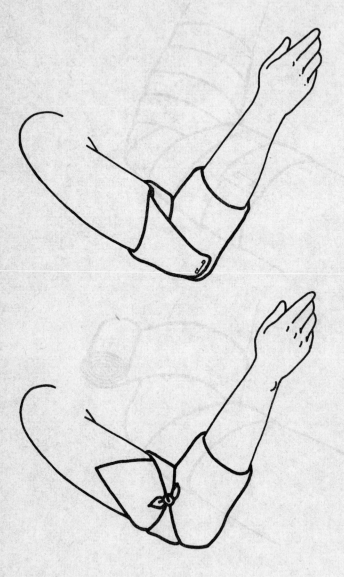

ELBOW BANDAGE / BANDAGE DU COUDE

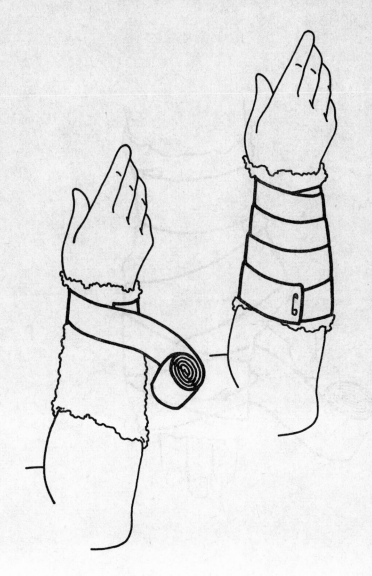

ROLLER BANDAGE : FOREARM / BANDAGE CIRCULAIRE - AVANT -BRAS

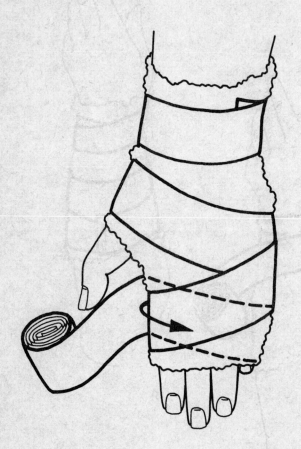

ROLLER BANDAGE : HAND / BANDAGE CIRCULAIRE - MAIN

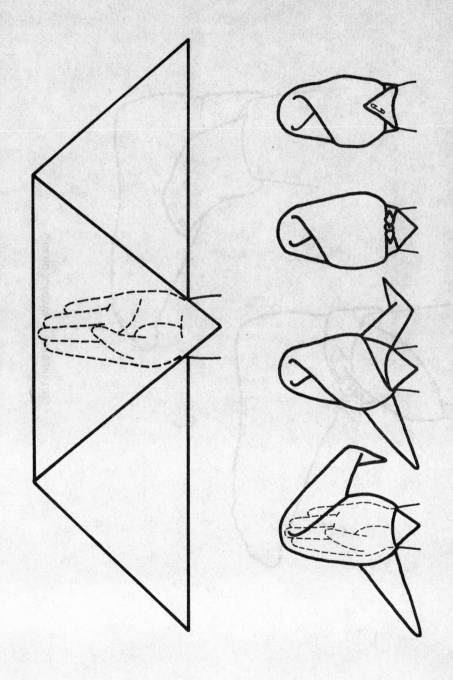

HAND BANDAGE / BANDAGE DE LA MAIN

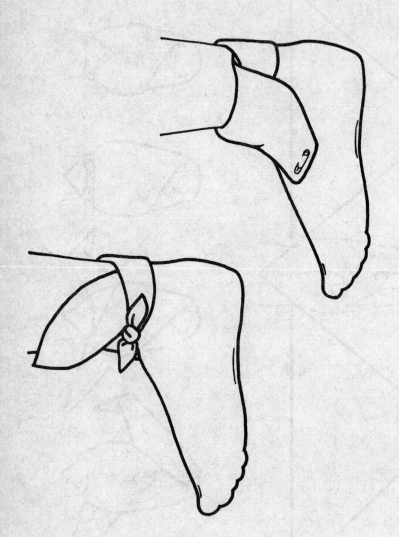

FOOT BANDAGE / BANDAGE DU PIED

5.   <u>COUNTING THE PULSE</u>

1.   Have a watch with a second-hand in front of you.

2.   Place two fingers of your right hand above the patient's wrist as indicated on the drawing.

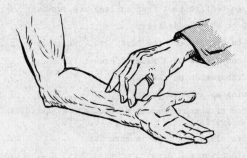

3.   Press very slightly. You should feel a regular beat; this is the pulse.

4.   Count it for a full minute looking at your watch: the number of beats you count in one minute is the pulse rate.

Normally it is between 70 and 80 per minute.

It increases with:

- effort (so take the pulse when the patient has rested)
- fever ($38^{o}C$ = around 100
          $39^{o}C$ = around 120)
- dehydration (a pulse rate of 130 without fever may be a sign of severe dehydration)
- some diseases of the heart.

6. <u>OTHER TECHNIQUES CAN BE FOUND IN THE TEXT AND ILLUSTRATIONS</u>:

ANATOMICAL   DIAGRAMS
(included here to help trainers with their instruction)

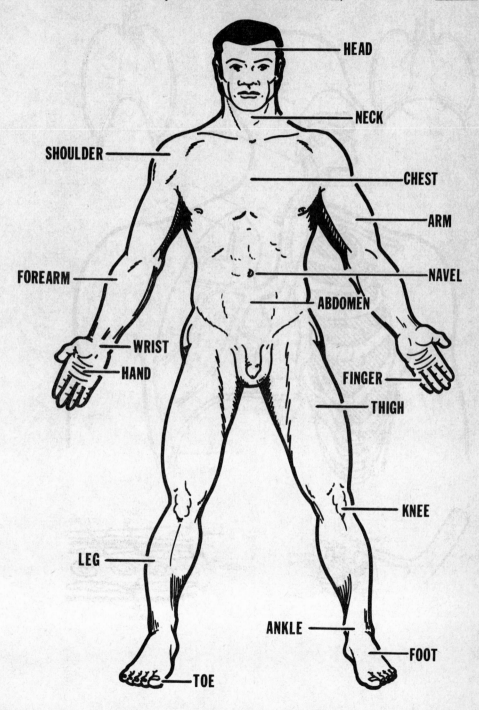

DIAGRAM OF THE RESPIRATORY SYSTEM

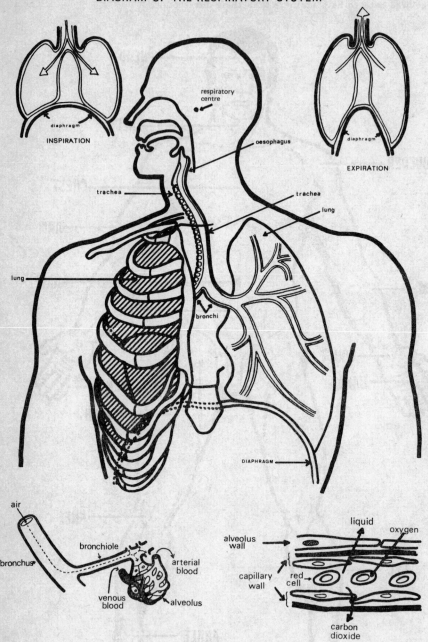

DIAGRAM OF THE CIRCULATORY SYSTEM

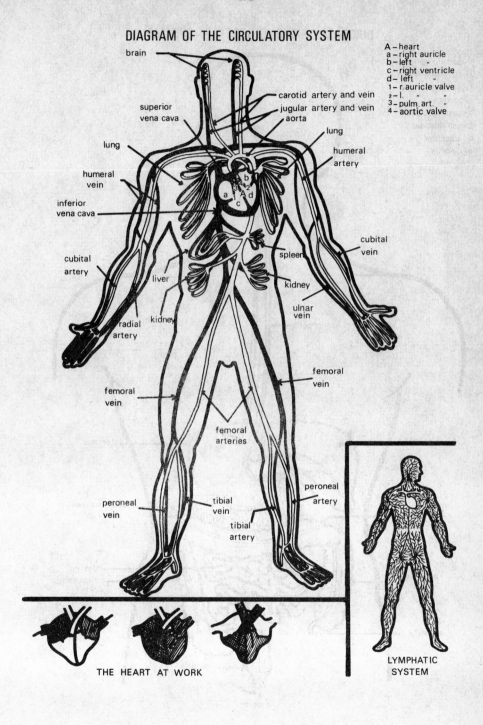

A – heart
a – right auricle
b – left   "
c – right ventricle
d – left   "
1 – r. auricle valve
2 – l.   "   "
3 – pulm. art.   "
4 – aortic valve

brain

carotid artery and vein
jugular artery and vein
aorta

superior vena cava

lung

humeral artery

lung

humeral vein

inferior vena cava

cubital vein

cubital artery

liver

spleen

kidney

radial artery

kidney

ulnar vein

femoral vein

femoral vein

peroneal artery

femoral arteries

peroneal vein

tibial vein

tibial artery

THE HEART AT WORK

LYMPHATIC SYSTEM

DIAGRAM OF THE DIGESTIVE SYSTEM

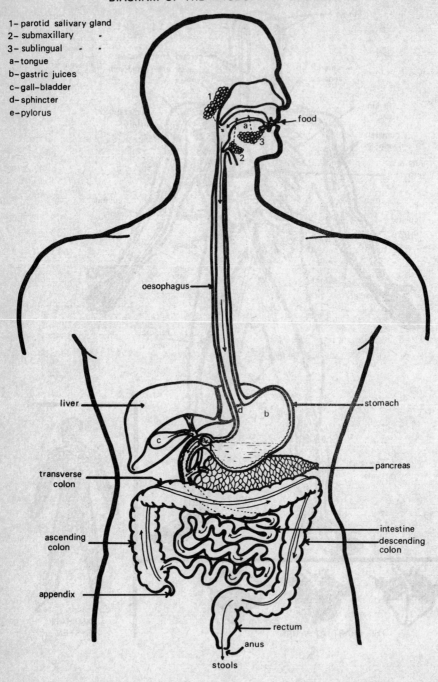

1– parotid salivary gland
2– submaxillary　　"
3– sublingual　　"　"
a– tongue
b– gastric juices
c– gall–bladder
d– sphincter
e– pylorus

food

oesophagus

liver

stomach

pancreas

transverse colon

intestine

ascending colon

descending colon

appendix

rectum

anus

stools

DIAGRAM OF THE URINARY SYSTEM

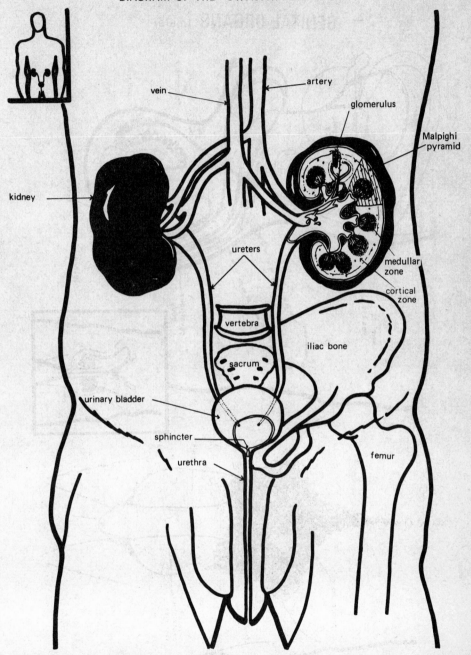

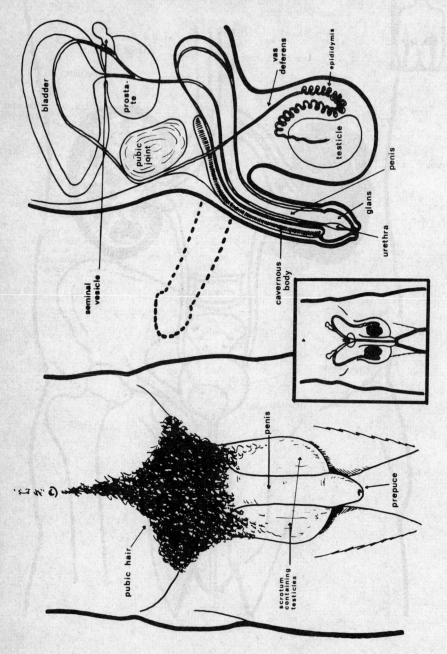

GENITAL ORGANS (male)

bladder

prosta-
te

pubic
joint

vas
deferens

epididymis

testicle

penis

glans

urethra

seminal
vesicle

cavernous
body

penis

prepuce

pubic hair

scrotum
containing
testicles

GENITAL ORGANS (female)

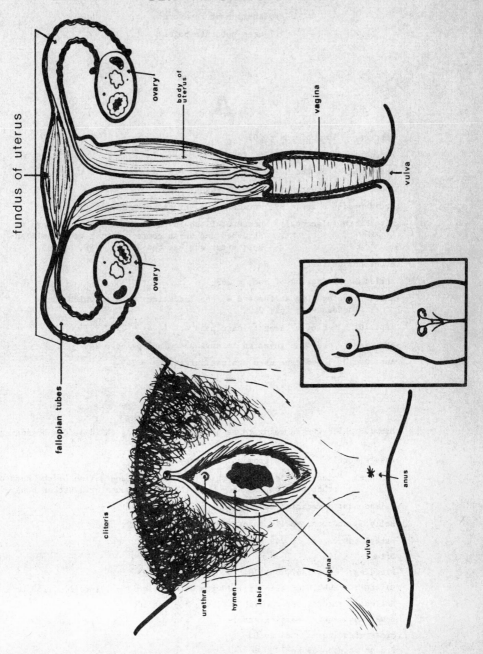

INDEX / GLOSSARY

with

explanation of key words

(figures refer to pages)

A

Abscess: lump of pus - 209

Abdomen: the belly - 174, 249

Abdominal: of the belly - 174, 249

Abortion: interruption of a pregnancy - 55

Accidents: burns - 99, wounds - 107, fractures - 117, bites - 123

Afterbirth (placenta):   piece of flesh in the womb to which the cord is attached and which comes out of a woman half an hour after she has had a baby - 55, 62, 63

After the delivery: - 64

Ankle: see drawing of body - 269

Anus: the opening at the end of the intestines through which one defecates - 252, 253

Aspirin: medicine taken to ease pain and fever - 249

Atropine: medicine injected to ease abdominal pains - 249

Aureomycin: medicine used against infections - 249

B

Baby: child who is going to be born; a very young child before beginning to walk

Baby's bottle: bottle from which a baby drinks

Bandage: piece of clean cloth which is wrapped round a limb or the head or other part of the body when there is a wound or a broken bone - 259-266

Belladonna: medicine used to ease pains in the belly - 249

Belly: abdomen. Belly pains: - 53, 82, 174, 189, 249

Benzyl benzoate: - 249

Bites: - 123

Bleeding: - 44, 67, 76, 78, 79, 107 to 116, 197

Blister: bubble on skin filled with watery liquid - 101 to 103, 158 to 159

Boiled: said of water which has been kept at 100°C

Bowel movement: passing stools

Breast-feeding: - 84 to 88

Breast pain: 69 to 70

Burns: - 99 to 106

Buttocks: the flesh on the backside - 254

C

Chest: see drawing of body - 269

Childbirth: birth of a baby - 54 to 63

Chloroquine: medicine used against infections, fevers - 249

Chlorpromazine: medicine used in mental disorders - 249

Cholera: communicable disease with diarrhoea, vomiting and dehydration
           which occurs in large epidemics - 20

Coil: kind of contraceptive - 76 to 78

Communicable diseases: diseases which can be transmitted from one person
                         to another. Example: measles, tuberculosis - 10 to 42

Community development: social activity in which members of a community meet to
                         discuss their common needs, suggest answers and implement
                         action - 220 to 237

Compresses: piece of clean cloth used for dressing a wound or for soothing an
              itch or a pain - 111 to 112, 161, 169, 209

Condom: kind of contraceptive; a sheath - 75, 76

Conjunctiva: the part of the eye that is normally white

Constipation: difficulty in defecating or the passing of hard stools - 67

Consultation: visit by a patient

Contraceptives: means of preventing pregnancy - 74 to 78

Convulsions: violent involuntary movements - 14 to 15, 53, 216 to 219

Cord: cord which joins a baby to its mother - 60 to 62

Cough: - 25 to 31, 39, 41

Cure: to restore to health, or recovery from an illness

D

Defecate: to pass stools (see stool), have a bowel movement - 136 to 141

Dehydration: when someone has lost a lot of water from his body (in diarrhoea,
               for instance) and needs to replace the water - 17, 20

Delivery: - 54 to 63

Diarrhoea: passing at least three liquid stools a day - 16 to 24, 39, 177

Discharge: yellowish liquid (for instance, from the nose, the ear, the eye,
             the penis or vagina) - 29, 30, 34 to 36, 80, 169

Diseases of women: - 79 to 83

Disinfect: to clean so as to protect against infection

Dress: put a dressing on a wound or limb

Dressing: piece of clean cloth used to cover a wound or burn - 103, 105, 108, 113

E

e.g.:   "for example"

Enema: injection of liquid into the anus

Epidemic: when several people catch the same disease about the same time - 37 to 42

Ergotamine: medicine used for bleeding after delivery or miscarriage - 250

Excreta: stools (see stool)

Excreta disposal: - 135 to 141

Eyelid: the pieces of skin above and below the eye that partly cover it - 166 to 169

Eye diseases: - 163 to 169

F

Faeces: stools (see stool)

Family welfare: - 73 to 78

Fertilizer: substance or product that makes corn or vegetables grow better - 227

Fever: body temperature higher than $37.5°C$ - 11 to 15

Feverish: said of a patient who is not well and whose temperature is over $37.5°C$

Flushes, hot flushes: - 82

Fodder: dried grass, straw, hay, etc. for feeding cattle

Foodstuffs: substances used as food, something that people eat - 224 to 231

Forceps: special instrument for holding objects;   surgical pincers

Forearm: see drawing of body - 269

Fracture: broken bone - 117 to 122

G

Genital: of the sex organs

Genitals: sex organs

Gentian violet: liquid to put on skin for cleaning wounds - 250

Germs: very small living animals which attack the human body. They can be seen only with a powerful glass or microscope - 10, 13, 86

Growth chart: - 90, 91

H

Handicapped person: a person who cannot use the arms, hands or legs in a normal way, or a person who cannot learn like other people

Headaches: - 53, 170 to 173

Hygiene: cleanliness; healthy habits

I

i.e.: "that is to say"

Incision: to make an incision: to cut, to open with a blade

Infection: when a germ enters the body or the skin and multiplies. It may produce fever, pain, diarrhoea, coughing, redness, pus or other discharge

Injection: liquid put into the buttock or the arm with a needle and syringe - 254 to 258

Intestinal worms: - 185 to 191

Iodine tincture: liquid put on skin for cleaning wounds - 250

Iron sulfate: medicine used against weakness after a lot of bleeding and in certain kinds of malnutrition - 250

J

Joint: the part joining two bones, e.g. the knee or the ankle - 179 to 184

L

Labour: the process of giving birth - 55

Latrine: dug hole into which stools are dropped - 136 to 141, 190

Learning objective: what a PHW should know or be able to do after he has studied a problem or practised a skill and which he did not know or could not do before

Lumps: 205 to 211

M

Malnutrition: being underfed or fed with the wrong foods - 93 to 98

Maternal care: - 43 to 83

Medicines: drugs - 248 to 251

Mepacrine: medicine taken to get rid of flatworms - 250

Mental disorders: - 212 to 219

Microscope: an instrument with which we can see germs and other objects that are too small to be seen with our eyes alone

Miscarriage: delivery of a baby before it can live outside the womb - 55, 63, 250

Mortar: mixture of sand, cement and water

Mouth: diseases of the mouth - 198 to 204

Mouth-to-mouth resuscitation: a way of reviving someone who seems dead - 92

Mucus: thick liquid, slime produced inside the body - 22

N

Nasal: of the nose

Navel: see drawing of body - 269

Nutrition: - 84 to 98

O

Objective: see Learning objective

Ocular: of the eye

Ointment: medicine in the form of a paste to apply on skin (or in some cases on eyes) - 167, 168, 249

Ophthalmic: of the eye

Oral rehydration salts: packet of powder to dissolve in drinking water for making the oral fluid used to treat diarrhoea

Oxytocin: medicine injected to stop bleeding quickly after delivery or miscarriage - 250

P

Pains in the joints: - 179 to 184

Pap: semi-liquid food for infants, mash - 88

Penicillin: medicine used against infections - 251

Penis: the male sex organ

Period: loss of blood from below (vagina) that a woman has every month - 43, 79, 80, 82, 83, 178

Phenobarbital: medicine used to calm excited persons, or help them to sleep - 251

Pill: round piece of medicine. Special pills are used as contraceptives

Piperazine: medicine taken against round or small worms - 251

Placenta: see Afterbirth - 55, 62, 63

Postnatal care: - 64 to 72

Pregnancy: when a woman is expecting a baby - 43 to 53

Pregnant woman: woman who is expecting a baby - 43

Procaine penicillin: a kind of penicillin. See Penicillin - 251

Purgative: medicine taken to make it easier to pass stools

Pulse: heart beats felt at an artery, usually at the wrist - 20, 267

Pus: yellowish liquid that comes out of an infected wound - 166, 208, 209

R

Records: - 238 to 241

Red spots: - 29, 30, 36, 158, 159

Refer: send to the nearest hospital or health centre

Refuse: rubbish, dirt or waste that is thrown away

Rehydration: replacing the water lost from the body when dehydration occurs
(especially in diarrhoea) - 20, 21

Reports: - 242 to 248

Respiratory disease: - 25 to 31

Rubbish: refuse, dirt or waste that is thrown away

Runny nose: - 25 to 31

S

Scab: small piece of hard dry skin - 158 to 162

Sexual intercourse: when a man and woman come together sexually

Sexually-transmitted diseases: - 32 to 36

Sheath: a cover used as contraceptive - 75, 76

Skin disease: - 155 to 162

Skinfold: crease in the skin - 19

Spitting: - 25 to 31

Splint: piece of wood or other material used to support a broken leg
or arm - 120, 121

Spots: see red spots

Sputum: coughed-up matter - 25, 26

Sticking plaster: piece of clean cloth which sticks and is used to hold
dressings and close a wound - 11, 113 to 115

Stiff: rigid; not flexible. Stiff neck - 172

Stool: what the body passes out through the anus, faeces

Stretcher: bed carried by two people to carry a sick person - 233

Sulfadiazine: medicine taken against infections - 251

Sunken eyes: the eyes fall back into the skull (= a sign of dehydration) -
19, 20

Supervisor: person who comes at intervals to give you advice, and to whom
you are responsible

Swallow: to pass food or drink down the throat

Swelling: enlargement of a limb or of part of a limb. May also be a small
bump or lump under the skin - 51, 52, 72, 95 to 97, 173, 182, 194, 195

Syringe: instrument for giving injections - 258

T

Tablet: flat piece of medicine - 248 to 251

Techniques: - 252 to 268

Teeth - Diseases of teeth: - 198 to 204

Temperature: internal heat of the body, that can be measured with a
thermometer. 37°C = normal. Above 37.5°C = fever.
Above 39°C = high temperature - 252, 253

Tetracycline: medicine used against certain infections - 24, 251

Thigh: see drawing of body - 269

Tiredness: - 83, 111, 192 to 197, 211, 215

Transport and communication: - 232 to 237

U

Ulcer: an open sore

Urinate: to pass water

Uterus: see womb

V

Vaccination: a means of protecting the body against germs which may
enter it - 10

Vagina)
Vulva) :   female genitals

Vegetable oil: oil which comes from plants

Venereal diseases: - 32 to 36

Vomiting: - 15, 31, 38, 41, 44, 48, 52, 96, 175, 176, 189

W

Waste disposal: - 142 to 148

Water supply: - 129 to 135

Weakness: - 83, 111, 192 to 197, 215

Welfare: well-being

Womb: pouch in which a baby grows inside the mother - 43

Worms: parasites (small animals) living in the belly (or under the
skin) - 185 to 191

Wound: where the skin is torn or broken; the flesh may or may not
be deeply cut - 107 to 116

Wrist: see drawing of the body - 269

PART II

★

Guidelines

for

training PHWs

★★★

Introduction

Learners and teachers are both engaged in an exciting experience. To begin with, let us not think of the "teacher" as the person who knows everything and the "learner" as one who knows little or nothing. We all "know" something which can be shared, and in this way we learn from each other. There are principles and methods which can make learning stimulating, interesting and useful. This, Part II, discusses and outlines some of these principles and methods. It does not discuss WHAT should be taught but HOW the teaching/learning can best be done. It is intended mainly to help instructors, supervisors and primary health workers to use and teach the content of Part I of this book. It may be used also as reference material to prepare local manuals adapted to local needs. However, we should stress that the order in which the problems in Part I are selected to be taught may differ from one situation to the other. In one country it may be necessary and possible to teach all the problems. In another country, students may be able to learn only a few problems at a time or only a few priority problems, some of which may be mentioned in Part I. The programme will be longer in some situations than in others. Students may learn to deal with a few problems and then work in the community for a while; they may then be recalled to learn to deal with more problems, or they may learn to deal with many problems with no interruption. Learning does not start at a fixed time and end at another fixed time - it is a continuous process throughout life.

Part II is organized in four chapters. It starts by discussing the kind of knowledge and information that is basic to any training programme, and it goes on to describe some methods and techniques for making learning/teaching more effective; then it describes how to assess whether the training has achieved its purposes. It ends with examples of how to organize learning modules, starting from the statement of a problem and going on to what the student will be able to do, and whether he has learned what he is expected to learn.

1.

Getting to know

each other

Before we begin training we should first create a harmonious working atmosphere. We need to ask ourselves: Who are the students? Where have they come from? What have they been doing in their family, their community? Who is the teacher? Where has he come from? What is his background? Becoming acquainted with one another is very important for successful learning. Teachers can encourage this by presenting themselves, their experience, where they come from, etc. Students can be invited to do the same. Seats can be arranged in a circle so that students can talk <u>with</u> each other instead of looking at the teacher only.

There may be entrance requirements which describe the minimum qualifications students need in order to join the programme (e.g. primary school - read and write the local language - age, etc.). However, encouraging students to talk about their own backgrounds is another way of finding out more about them. At the same time, students and teachers can share and compare their experience and voice their expectations of the programme. This period of adjustment, the orientation period, may last for a few days or even more. Obviously the kind of background from which a student comes, his role in the family and community, and his general approach and attitude to learning, will influence very much the length of the training, the kind of language used, and what he gains from the training.

Summary: Learning process

Learning process	
Method (How)	Content (What)

- Getting to know
  each other
	- Working Guide for
	  Primary Health
	  Workers:
	  Introduction, page 3
	  The Primary Health
	  Worker profile

2.

Suggested techniques

for

making learning / teaching

useful, realistic and effective

1. GETTING TO KNOW THE COMMUNITY

We receive much of our education from our surroundings - where we live, our
family and society. We learn direct from our own experience and indirectly from
others. We compare what we already know with what we learn during training. To
understand how a community works what could be better than to discuss the community
from which the students come? Talking about the community is how the discussion starts.
How does the community work? Who are its leaders? Why are these people leaders?
Who has influence? Why? What makes a family - what are its problems and needs?
What are the traditions and customs? Who takes care of people when they are sick?
How do families work together for each other or for the community? Who in the family
decides what a family should do? Who decides what a community should do? How can
these people help the PHW? What must the PHW do to obtain their help? What would
happen if he did not get their support?

In order to understand the community very well, we need to work in it. Here
are some suggestions: students can be divided into small groups of three to five;
each group can be given the task of finding out and showing with pictures and diagrams
what they know of the community: a group may be responsible for drawing a map showing
main roads and tracks, the main areas where people live, and the sites of the market,

school, community house, etc. Another group could be responsible for finding out
how many people live in a given area (the area may consist of many villages which
together make up a zone) or the number of children under five years of age. Practice
in counting the number of people or children is very important, as it helps us to do
the same later where we work. We can use the same method to find out, if asked to do
so, the number of women aged fifteen to forty-five years, and to record the number
of children born. Besides these, groups can ask other questions - for instance,
about:
- values, beliefs and customs of the community
- family system
- child-bearing practices

- attitudes towards health, knowledge about sickness, usual behaviour

- resources: - how people make money or get food
             - agriculture, crafts, services, animal husbandry, etc.
             - water/sanitation
             - roads/telephones/radios/electricity/transportation

- political structure

- main faith, religion

For each task a clear statement must be written of what the group has to do and
the time allowed in which to do it. The small groups share their findings with the
entire group so that a complete picture of the community is obtained. Finding out
the answers to these questions leads to a better understanding of the community.

A.   *FINDING OUT THE PROBLEMS OF THE COMMUNITY*

First, what is a problem? A problem is a situation or condition which causes
a difficulty or which is upsetting. It may occur in an individual, a family or
in the community. Something must be done to solve a problem or make it less serious.

Often, we find that we know or can feel that something is wrong, but do not
know why. Sometimes, we notice a problem which is not considered to be a problem
by the people concerned. However, it is sure that if something is upsetting a
person or a community, and if one listens carefully to what people say, and to the
needs they express, one will soon find out what they are concerned about. We need
to remind ourselves from time to time that we must let people speak for themselves;

we should not come to the community with ready-made solutions. Instead we can suggest possible or alternative actions to improve the situation. Learning how to deal with problems is a continuing process, and the more practical experience we get the better we can help the communities we serve. Thus, we can start developing these skills now. A few suggestions follow on how to go about it.

B. APPROACHING THE COMMUNITY

1. The teacher contacts the village authorities and, at their convenience, organizes with them a meeting with the student group. It may be more convenient for the village representatives to come to the training centre and discuss community organization with the students. Then, agreement to visit all families should be obtained so that the group gets first-hand experience with people in their homes.

2. Send the class in small groups into the community. Let them come back with a list of problems that they feel are the most important and that the community has said are important.

3. Each group visits a community of about forty families. The small group divides into pairs and plans how many families each pair will visit in order to cover the whole area. No more than two students should visit a household at one time.

4. A home visit may appear like an intrusion unless it is done properly; that is: the students introduce themselves to the family, explain who they are and why they are visiting, for example, to join in helping the people to help themselves. They should observe the conditions and circumstances of the family and obtain information by asking questions such as the following:

- where does the family come from? and why did it come to this area?

- how large is the family? (a family nucleus or an extended family?)

- how many children? and what do they do?

- have any children died? why? or what was the cause?

- what does the head of the family do to get money? or food? or seed? etc.

- what does the family eat? when do they eat? who prepares the food?

- has anyone in the family been sick during the past week - month? what did they do? where did they go?

- what is the general condition of the house?

- how big is the house?

- how many people share a room?

- are there windows/ventilation?

- do they have water and how do they store it?

- where do they get their water from? how far is it?

- is the food protected from flies, rats, etc.?

- how do they get rid of rubbish?

- is there a latrine? is it individual or collective? how well is it used
    and kept? if not, where do the members of the family defecate?

The information obtained should be written on a family record card.

This first community visit may take some time; working hours of the people, distance and transport all have to be thought about, but all other learning will be linked to the situation in the family and community. So it is worth while to spend enough time planning and making the visit at the beginning of the training. This will help to build good relations between the students and their teachers and between them and the communities they will serve. The student/teacher group will have a chance to discuss the problems found and the solutions suggested.

C. RANKING PRIORITIES

Since we cannot solve all the problems of a community we have to determine which are the most important. Thus, it is useful to list the problems according to how important the community sees them.

One way of determining how important the problems are is to find out how many people say something about the same problem. When students return from the community the number of times a problem has been stated is counted. This information can be put on the blackboard and soon it will be obvious which are the three or four problems that need immediate attention. For example:-

No water supply in the village (this may be said in many ways e.g. "a long way to fetch water")	50 families
No nearby health care clinic or none open at a suitable time (e.g. expressed as "we go to the hospital which is far away" or "the service is closed in the afternoon")	40 families

        Not enough food   25 families
        (e.g. expressed as "poor
        harvest, drought", etc.)

The most important problems listed are the <u>priority concerns of the community</u>.

    Let us suppose that a large number of people in the community agree that at that
moment the following five sets of problems are the most important: (i) problems
related to emergency and curative care; (ii) problems of water and sanitation;
(iii) problems of food; (iv) problems of work and money to buy things that are
needed; (v) problems of communications (no road, no radios, no bus, etc.).

    These five sets of problems <u>are only examples</u> of what a community might consider
important. Other communities may have different problems. Most of them will probably
concern food, housing, health (the community might say sickness), transportation to
markets or towns, and education (schooling for children).

    Coming back to our five sets of problems, it is obvious that it is impossible
for one person to do everything. This leads the group to ask the following questions:
what do we think we could do that would be most helpful to the community, and what
do we think we can do at the end of the training period? We should remind ourselves
that we must always <u>compare</u> what we learn and what we do <u>with the real situation</u>;
that is, where the problem actually is, in the home or the community. This is
important because people must understand whatever we do and say. What we do and
say must be practical for the people. For example, we cannot tell a mother to give
her child medicine at 8.00 a.m., 12.00 and 6.00 p.m., when she does not have a watch
or a clock, but we can tell her by the sun.

D.   *DECIDING TOGETHER WHAT IS TO BE DONE*

    Based upon the agreed role of the Primary Health Worker (see pages 3, 5, 339 and
340), students and teachers should discuss what they think they can do in and with
the community. One person could write down the different ideas and what the general
agreement is.

    For example, students might say they will be able:

    - to give medicine to the sick

    - to put a dressing on a wound

    - to deliver a baby

- to talk with the people about health

- to help children not to get sick.

These and other tasks we should like to do, which can be listed, are tasks we shall learn how to do. For others we shall have to learn to seek the help of other people working in the community. If students list tasks that cannot be done the teacher must explain why they are not possible.

2. LEARNING TO WORK WITH OTHERS

There is always something a person can do for himself (or a mother can do for her child) to alleviate a problem. The PHW may be able to teach people to do some things for themselves. But the PHW can only do what he is trained to do, and if he is unable to solve a problem he seeks the help of others who know what to do. If it is an illness it may be the nurse or medical assistant; if it is about drought or a poor harvest, it may be the village council, a community development officer or an agricultural officer; if it is a dirty well it will be the health inspector or sanitarian. This way of working with others is called teamwork; it is necessary because the various people such as the sanitarian, the agricultural officer and others know something different from what we know, and we can share this together since we are working for the same goal. To do our share we must understand the health problems and learn certain skills.

Summary: Learning about the community

Learning process	
Method (How)	Content (What)
- Approaching the community - Finding out the problems of the community - Ranking priorities	- Getting to know the community - Priority concerns of the community, deciding together what is to be done (see role of the PHW, pages 3, 5, 339 and 340)

3. <u>SETTING OUT WHAT WE NEED TO LEARN AND HOW TO LEARN IT</u>

Let us look at the five problems discussed on page 292, which can be related to the problems in Part I. We will need to know:

(a) What does the person feel (pain, worry, discomfort) and what does
     he show? (red spots on the face, swollen legs, etc.);

(b) What has caused this problem or what started it? Usually there is
     more than one cause, e.g. a child is very hot and is coughing. He
     coughs because germs have gone into his chest; he becomes more ill
     because he is very thin and does not have enough to eat and drink;

(c) When we have learnt the cause we must ask how the problem could have
     been prevented or what could have been done so that the problem
     might have been less severe;

(d) What do people do for this problem? or, what are the usual remedies?
     is this enough or what else can we do?

There are some things that people do to cure the problem. There are other things that people can do to make sure the problem is less likely to start (this is called <u>prevention</u>; or, we say, people can <u>prevent</u> a problem).

When we have this information, we can talk about what is a normal condition. For example, a person who is never sick, who eats well and eats enough of the right kind of food, who is strong and able to work and learn well is said to be in normal health. The child who has a cough is not in a normal condition; the normal condition is when he is not coughing; it is also when he eats well and his height and weight are right for his age.

After we discuss the normal condition, we can talk about how the normal condition can be kept up, and what are the first signs that something is wrong; what can be done to prevent it from becoming more serious; what can be done if more care is needed. To do this we must break down the problem into small parts.

A.   BREAKING DOWN THE PROBLEM INTO SMALL PARTS

Each problem can be broken down into several parts to make it easier for us to know what to do, step by step, why to do it and when to do it. For example, if we take <u>Problem 1.3</u> in Part I: "<u>Diarrhoea</u>", we have to know the following:-

- whether it is diarrhoea
- what other signs and symptoms there are
- how serious it is
- what treatment to give
- what advice to give
- should we refer the problem

In order to know this the PHW should be able to:

1. Ask the person, or the mother of a child: How many times did you (or
    the child) pass stools? What were they like? Did they cause you pain?
    How long have you had loose stools? What did you eat for your last
    meal? What did you drink?

2. Examine the patient to see if the eyes are sunken, the mouth dry, and
    the tongue dry and red; if upon pinching the skin the crease remains;
    if the pulse is difficult to feel.

3. Do the following:
        take the temperature, and
        examine stools for blood and mucus

4. Treat the condition as described in Problem 1.3.

5. Advise and instruct as needed.

In order to do all the above we have to learn how to:

- ask questions and listen
- write down the answers briefly
- examine a person
- take the temperature and pulse
- examine stools
- prepare liquid solution if ready-made packages are not available
- decide which treatment to give and when to refer the patient to the hospital
    or health centre
- teach a person to prepare the liquid solution and when and how to give or
    take it
- advise on prevention of diarrhoea - need for personal hygiene, for food
    hygiene (flies, water, etc.)

These actions are examples of learning objectives; that is, what you set out
to learn and should be able to do at the end of your training.

Each step takes time to learn. For example, it may take a few hours to learn
to ask questions and listen to answers, and ten or more hours to be able to do this
well. It may take several hours to learn to take the pulse accurately. The group
can practise these skills on each other. This applies also to taking the temperature.
It is important to take the necessary time to learn well.

Problems are linked together. Once these are learned they may be used in many
different situations. For example, you will need to ask questions of a person who
coughs - you will need to examine him, take the temperature and pulse, give treatment
and advice. If he is not complaining of diarrhoea you will know that you do not have
to examine the stools or prepare dehydration fluid but you may need to do other tasks.
Every problem can be broken down into smaller problems and by doing so learning is
made easier.

By following this method it will be seen that some procedures for dealing with
one problem may be used to solve another problem; therefore, we do not necessarily
have to follow the order in which problems are presented in Part I. We may choose
to learn first a particular problem because it is a priority concern of the community.
This we have already discussed when we were finding out problems of the community and
ranking them according to priority.

B.   *EXAMPLES OF HOW TO TEACH AND LEARN DIFFERENT PARTS OF A PROBLEM*

Once we have broken down a problem, we can use different methods for learning
about the different parts of the problem. Some examples are:

(a) Group method: Some things are better learned in groups. When we talked
about approaching the community we described how to use a small group for interviewing.
Before small groups perform a task, they should receive clear instructions which should
be understood by everyone. After small groups have finished the task, they should come
together again in a large group to talk about what the groups have done and to find out
if and how it could be done better.

(b) Do-it-yourself methods: Sometimes, we need to seek information by ourselves,
e.g. by reading or asking questions of someone outside class, or practising a skill
alone after it has been demonstrated with others.

(c) Demonstration method: Some skills can be taught by showing the whole group
or small groups how a task is performed and then asking one or two people to repeat
it. Everyone should have a chance to practise individually. This is a good method of
learning a manual skill, for example, giving an injection or delivering a baby.

(d) <u>Story-telling</u>: Another method is to make up a story using three or four ideas. This is a good way of making sure that what is learned makes sense to people.

(e) <u>Play-acting</u>: The group can make up a play or drama about three or four ideas, as with story-telling. In countries where puppets are traditional, this is also a good method.

(f) <u>Use of proverbs, jokes, songs and dances</u>: These methods can also help to explain ideas. They can use the language of the students.

(g) <u>Use of pictures, posters, diagrams</u>: Some things are learned better when people can <u>see</u> rather than just hear about something. Pictures, posters and diagrams are called <u>visual aids</u>, and they are useful for learning.

(h) <u>Questioning</u>: We can ask the group questions or ask them to ask questions after other methods have been used, to make sure that everyone has understood and is clear about what has been taught.

C.   ENJOYING LEARNING

Here we suggest ways of making learning and teaching more active and interesting. They can be used in many different situations and by teachers with students or the PHW with community groups.

A wise man has said that in life we need to want to do what we have to do. We have to want to do what people need us to do in our work and daily life. The meaning of this is very simple: we can enjoy learning and working if we set our minds and hearts on them.

How can we develop this feeling in ourselves and in others? Here are some suggestions:

- We have already some reason for wanting to learn because we came to the training programme. Many things may have helped us; for example, our elders may have encouraged us to join the programme. Since we have come, visits to the community and talking about its problems have shown us we can help our neighbours and the community. When we see that what we learn will be useful in our work, we enjoy or look forward to learning. The role of the teacher here is very important - he should know that learning cannot be forced. Students learn in different ways and at different rates; therefore, do not have a fixed schedule, a fixed time and a fixed experience for all. The teacher should also know that students learn better when they are motivated and satisfied, and when they take an active part in learning, in conditions

like those in which they will be working later. Therefore he must encourage
students to learn by organizing visits to the community, by talking about students'
future work and the problems they will face. Equally important is the teacher's
attitude - when he shows interest and enthusiasm he helps the students to become
interested and enthusiastic also, and they may adopt this attitude. Students of
teachers who enjoy teaching not only enjoy learning but also learn better and
remember what they have learned; this is partly because one teaches what one is,
and not only what one knows.

- We must make sure that what we say, what we do and what we think make sense
in real life. This point has already been made but must always be kept in mind.
One way is to ask questions; this stimulates discussion and helps students to
relate the teaching to their own experience. Another way of keeping in touch
with reality is to use anecdotes, folklore and local jokes: in one country, it
is said of a self-important person who tries to do unpopular things that "his
head is too big for his hat" and in another country that "he strains to leave
droppings as big as an elephant's". A touch of humour makes learning more
lively.

- We can encourage students to ask questions about what they have not
understood; and to show what they have understood by specific examples. What is
not understood must be gone over immediately until it is clear to everybody. This
will lead to a sense of achievement. Everyone will feel proud that everything has
been understood. There is nothing more frustrating than not understanding and not
being helped to understand; or being unable to do something and not being helped
to learn how to do it. Once we understand or know how to perform a task it is
important to show in some way what we have understood and make sure that we have
understood it correctly.

- Reward is one of the best ways of helping students to learn. When we
feel that what we do is useful, and this is recognized and appreciated by others,
we feel pleased. Students need to be encouraged. We can praise their efforts,
their creative ideas, initiative and hard work. Punishment upsets people. If
we make fun of a student or rebuke him in front of others, he may not enjoy

- 299 -

learning. Sometimes, we have to fail a student in an examination, but we should encourage him afterwards so that he does not later learn only for fear of being punished. A common saying in some countries is "if you are bitten by a snake you become afraid of a rope".

The teacher can reward students by making them realize that their efforts will lead to the well-being and development of the community. Also, he can sometimes invite community leaders to talk with the students so that they hear the community's point of view.

Summary: Setting out what we need to learn

Learning process	
Method (How)	Content (What)

- Breaking down the problem into small parts
 	
- Using different <u>methods</u>:
  - group
  - do-it-yourself
  - demonstration
  - story-telling
  - play-acting
  - jokes, songs, dances, proverbs
  - visual aids
  - questioning
 	
- Enjoying learning
	- Problems Nos. 4, 6, 5, 3, 7 in Part I
	
	- Enjoying learning

D.   EXAMPLES OF HOW TO USE DIFFERENT LEARNING/TEACHING METHODS

We must be careful to select the best methods. The methods used should depend
upon the problem to be solved and what has to be learned (see the learning objectives
listed at the beginning of each problem in Part I). Some problems are better handled
by group methods; for example, community development problems, where group decision
and action are necessary. Other problems are better taught individually, especially
when individual skills (e.g. manual skills) are being learned. Sometimes it is
better to use a few methods for learning about one problem or a group of problems
i.e. a combination of methods.

The students may meet as a whole group, e.g. during a film or demonstration, or
in small groups. Each group can be given a specific task or problem which can be
shared by the whole group.

ILLUSTRATION, IN STEP FORM, OF GROUP METHOD

These steps are outlined to facilitate planning for learning and teaching;
however, they are flexible and the order of steps may vary with the different
learning experiences.

STEP I: Reasons for the choice of the method

Instead of using all methods to illustrate what steps to take, we take the
group method as an example. This is useful when the problem requires:-

- the views of all concerned to be shared

- the experience of all concerned to be shared

- the development of communication skills such as:
    listening carefully to what others say
    speaking clearly
    stimulating others to talk
    stimulating others to want to do something (take action)
    developing a feeling of confidence
    sharing decision-making
    sharing action

<u>STEP II</u>: Linking problems together: Grouping problems for particular
           method selected.

Certain problems from Part I can best be taught by dealing with them
together:

- how to have clean water

- how to find new kinds of food

- how to eliminate rubbish (garbage)

- how to protect foodstuffs

- how to deal with epidemics

- how to develop means of transport and communication

- how to organize the community for vaccination.

All these problems demand community participation. This is because it is
the every-day activities of people and the conditions of the community that cause,
or lead to, problems. Actions have to be taken by the community to solve and
prevent these problems.

<u>STEP III</u>: Preparing learning activities suitable for the problem

In preparing for learning and in selecting the methods it is important to
understand the problem beforehand. All information about the problem should be
put together. All material and/or equipment needed to make discussion and
learning easier should be put together. Different methods can be used for
each problem such as group-work, role-playing, etc.

As an example of group learning, or the small-group method, let us turn
to Part I, Problem 5.1, "Water Supply". People say that their problem is having
to travel long distances to fetch water, or having too little water for all
purposes - drinking, washing and irrigation.

STEP IV: Preparation for the class

Before the class

Review Problem 5.1, "Water Supply", in Part I. Study the diagrams; note why some show a bad water supply, others a better one, and others the best water supply. Write down the different steps in learning this problem. Decide on the methods you will use for each step.

STEP V: Breaking down the problem

What shall we know and be able to do at the end of the learning period. At the end of the learning period, one should be able to:

1. Find out about the place where the villagers go to get water for drinking and washing themselves.

2. Tell when water from a pond or river can be safe for drinking.

3. Recognize whether water from a spring or well is sufficiently protected to be safe for drinking.

4. Explain to the village authorities that diseases are caused by dirty water, and tell them how the villagers can get clean water.

5. Explain to the village authorities how the people can get clean water from a spring or a well.

6. Explain to the villagers what parts of the river should be used for drawing drinking water, for bathing and for watering livestock (making sure that the water is not contaminated by the village higher up).

Let us say that you have decided to use the small-group method and to use the community for learning and teaching. Groups of three or four students will work together and visit the village to collect the necessary information.

STEP VI: The class begins

Ask the whole group to look at Problem 5.1 in Part I, to read carefully what is written and to study the diagrams.

Ask the group what are all the things they could possibly know and be able to do when the classes on "How to have a clean water supply" are completed. Invite a student to write on the blackboard what the group states. You may add steps, which

you have previously written down, that the students have omitted, to ensure that
all the steps are followed. Make sure that everyone has a chance to ask questions
if there are things they do not understand.

Using the Working Guide, Part I, show what you have seen in the village(s)
and then use the diagrams in the Working Guide. Point out which type of water
the village uses. Ask if there is a well in the village.

Discuss in the group where the well is, how the people get the water
e.g. with pails, with goat-skin bags, with earthenware jugs, with a pump.

Write the different answers on the blackboard. This would show the various
types of water sources, and methods of collecting the water.

Then move on to ask what this water is used for. Examples of answers might
be: for drinking (by people and animals), to irrigate the fields, to bathe in,
to wash and feed animals. We may already know that people urinate and defecate
in this water. In this case, try to draw out from the group that the water is
also used as a place for human excretion. Then go on to say that water can be
a cause of illness because it is used for so many purposes, and therefore it is
not safe (we say that the water is contaminated). At this point we can refer
to Problem 1.3 in the Working Guide, "Diarrhoea", and explain how contaminated
water causes diarrhoea.

Discuss how to make water safe for drinking. Refer to Problem 5.1, water
from the river, point 2; water from a spring, point 3; water from a well,
point 4.

STEP VII: Assignment of tasks to students

1. Arrange for students, in groups of three, to visit water sources in a village
and to describe them and make suggestions for improving them. The teacher may
assist them by asking questions such as: where is the water located? how is it
collected? what is needed to make water safer for drinking?

2. Ask the students to draw simple posters showing the situation before and after,
according to their suggestions.

STEP VIII: Discussions and conclusions

If students recommend that certain community actions are necessary, such as
covering wells or digging a new one (the old one being badly constructed or badly
placed), let them say how they would contact the community leaders, how they would

lead a community to take action (see learning about the community). What outside
assistance (health inspector or sanitarian) would be needed?

If the students do not make these recommendations, make sure to stimulate them
by asking suitable questions. Community contact and action would include: whom to
see - what to say - how to say it - whom to contact for further help. For example:
should a well be dug? where? by whom? what is needed? who should help? what are
the features of a good well? what is a contaminated well? how is the water in a
well safe? how is it sited in relation to latrines?

One group of students could act or make a play of a conversation between
the village authorities and themselves. In this play they would explain what work
is needed to protect a spring or well. Another group of students could draw three
posters to show three different places where people should draw water for drinking.

The end of this topic would lead us to talk about other problems related to
water such as "Diarrhoea" and other diseases that are transmitted when the water
is not clean. The water becomes contaminated because people and animals urinate
and defecate in it or along its edges. People who drink or bathe in this dirty
water may become sick. One should be able to decide what to teach next, when
the students have raised questions or problems.

Follow the same steps for similar problems. After the problem of water, it
would make sense to follow with "where to defecate" (see Problem 5.2), and linked
with this is the construction of latrines.

Let us outline key points which we need to remember about where to defecate
and the building of latrines: why build a latrine? what diseases will be prevented
if there are latrines? how is a latrine constructed? how is it used and kept in
good order? Here again we need to know our role, and to whom we should turn for help
when the villagers are convinced they should build latrines. This is how we work
with others (e.g. village authorities and sanitarians) and this is very important.

Let us look again at how to use the essential points in preparing our class,
and do so in such a way that the PHW can use the same methods in his work with the
community.

Read Problem 5.2 in Part I of the Working Guide. Break down the problem into
small parts:

1. Review the problem with the village authorities
2. What are the diseases in the village that are caused by people defecating
   in fields or rivers?

3. How many houses in the village have latrines? How do they look?
    How are they used? Are they clean? Why did these families decide
    to use latrines? Why did others decide not to use latrines?

What do we need to know about the problem?

1. How are diseases spread through muddy water? What happens in the
    body?
2. What are the signs?
3. What can we do to treat them?
4. What can we do to prevent them?
5. How is a latrine constructed? Can we get help from sanitation
    services?
6. Who constructed the latrine?
7. What are the characteristics of a good latrine?
8. What is our role?
9. What are the reasons why people do not have latrines?
10. What are the best ways to persuade them to change their minds?
11. What are the steps that village people can take that would lead
    most families to build their own latrines?

To do those things we may need to:

- Visit the village. For this, the teacher must organize a meeting with the
  village authorities.

- During the visit, try to find out how many families have latrines. The
  group should outline the information needed (as mentioned above).

- Review all the information, after we have answered questions 1 to 11; we
  can then prepare a story on how one of the diseases spreads and how the
  disease could be prevented by people using latrines. This story could
  be used by the PHW in the village when trying to persuade people to
  build latrines and PREVENT their becoming ill. The PHW could use
  information collected from the villagers themselves to make the stories
  REAL (e.g. reason for wanting to build a latrine). (See method how to
  use story-telling and role-playing).

STORY-TELLING

For thousands of years people have used stories to teach and to give examples of
beliefs, customs, and what they know of life. These stories have been, and continue

to be, transmitted from one generation to another, and have been very important in teaching people how to behave in certain situations. For example, mothers always teach their children how to behave with their elders, what to believe when faced with a problem, and what to do. This method of teaching is already in use and is very effective. So we can use it ourselves to transmit ideas and influence people to do what is necessary when faced with a problem. We should remember also that there may be traditional story-tellers in the village, and we should learn to give them facts to use in their story-telling, and learn from them how to go about telling a story.

If we learn how to prepare a story and tell it to others, we can then do the same when teaching others. When we listen to stories and find out what they mean, we can learn the causes and prevention of disease.

Developing a story

We must decide what we are going to talk about. As we develop the story we must imagine that we are in our community. We must write it as we would tell it to the community people. So we must know:-

- To whom are we going to tell the story?
- What are the two or three most important points that you want the listener to know? You should not include too many ideas, because the listener becomes confused.
- That the story should not be too long - and we should avoid including too many details.

For example, if we take the problem "The badly-fed child" (Problem 3.2 in Part I), the main points might be:

1.   The child is too thin because he does not eat enough or the right kind of food.
2.   The child is thin because he has diarrhoea.
3.   We can help to cure his sickness.
4.   We can help to prevent his sickness.
5.   We can discuss with the mother how she could give more or better food to her child.

Making up the story

Now we begin to make up a story to explain these ideas. Let us illustrate point 2: The child is thin because he has diarrhoea.

All children with diarrhoea are not in the same situation and you should
stress different things according to the situation you find. You must have stories
which suit the age of the person and perhaps how the disease shows itself. It is
best to use as your example how the disease is most usually caught, or the most
common practice or custom which leads to the illness. You must therefore ask
yourself as you put your story together "what is it that people do which causes
this particular illness?". The first example of a story could be about a child
with diarrhoea.

"The story begins when the mother goes to her weekly visit to the market.
Before leaving she tells her four children she has prepared some food for them,
which she has left on the mat. She tells them she might be late and to eat their
food when they want it. It is a very hot day and flies that have been walking
about on the rubbish heap have now sat on the food. Their feet are sticky and
dirty, and as they hop over the food they leave tiny germs which the children
cannot see, but which cause disease.

"The children eat their meal. They are very hungry and eat up all the
food, over which tiny germs are now scattered. The youngest, a weak and thin
little boy, sticks his fingers in the food and sucks them happily.

"During the night the little boy wakes and cries. He has a pain in his
tummy and passes a very loose stool. He passes several stools during the night
and in the morning is very miserable. Because the mother believes he will become
worse if he eats or drinks, she gives him no food or drink. For the next day or
two the little boy, already thin and frail, looks sad, his eyes sink in his head,
his skin is dry and loose and is creased like paper. Indeed, the poor little boy
looks more like an old man."

Talking about the story

At this point you may wish to ask the listeners questions: "what does that
story mean? what happened? why? what made the boy sick? why did his brothers
and sisters not become so sick?". You want to be sure that the students understand
that because the boy was already thin and frail he was too weak to fight the germs
that entered his body with the food. He lost a lot of water from his body in the
stools, and the water was not replaced because the mother believed she should give
him nothing to drink. You may wish at this point to continue with this story or

to tell a different story, about a well-fed child (see pages 84 to 92). This
story would tell how a well-fed child who gets diarrhoea recovers quickly
because:-

(a) he is already healthy - his height and weight are normal for
his age, and he is therefore strong

(b) he eats enough of the right kind of food

(c) his mother has learned from the PHW how to prepare food and drink,
and give them to her child in case of diarrhoea.

You may wish here to bring in other points which the mother may have learned
later from the PHW, e.g. always to cover food to protect it from flies and other
insects, and to burn rubbish or bury it away from the house. This could introduce
the problem of waste disposal (Problem No. 5.3 in the Working Guide) and you
could build another story around that.

We can see how one problem is linked to another and how one story can be
linked to another. To make sure that listeners have understood the meaning of
the story, you can ask questions about what happened and explain why it happened.
You can also ask students to repeat the stories in their own words or make up
other stories with the same meaning.

PLAY-ACTING

You may wish to suggest to students that they compose a play in which they
would act the different roles. The main points to be brought out must be explained.
The teacher can suggest plays and how the parts (roles) might be acted. In a big
class, small groups might each compose its own play. A group could do this one
day or evening, and present it next day to the whole class.

USE OF PROVERBS, JOKES, SONGS AND DANCES

Like story-telling, proverbs, jokes, songs and dances are part of every
culture and can be very useful for telling stories and conveying messages.
There may be proverbs, jokes, and even songs and dances that tell us about
health.

New jokes and songs can be prepared by groups as homework; they should
explain parts of a problem and solutions. The group should select good jokes
and songs which everyone likes and they should use them in teaching the community.

Many dances have special meanings for people even if some of the meanings have been forgotten. However, the PHW with people from the community could create dances with symbolic meaning about health and health practices, which could be explained at the time of the dance.

Puppet shows are a very lively way of stimulating interest and may be popular in your area. They can be used to act out a play or comedy.

DEVELOPING MANUAL SKILLS

Up to now we have been discussing problems and how we can learn. We have used a variety of methods in small or large groups. However, we all need to learn to do things by ourselves and we need to feel sure that we use our brains and hands together. Once we have learned the correct movements, the more we practise the better we become. These skills are mainly manual; this means we use our hands in order to do them. What are some of these skills? Examples are: giving an injection, delivering a baby, taking a temperature, putting on splints, making a stretcher, making solutions, putting drops in eyes and ears, examining a patient, etc. These are the main skills used in our daily work.

Each of these may be demonstrated. But we can say we have learned this particular skill only when we demonstrate that we have understood why we are doing it, and how we can do it. We must use certain instruments and equipment for each technique and we must become familiar with them so that we can use them smoothly, comfortably and safely.

Points to remember about demonstration

1. We must make sure that the group is not too large so that EVERYBODY can see what is done.

2. The students should always sit in a semi-circle, or half-moon. This is good for demonstration and group discussion.

3. Before we start the procedure we need to point out what equipment is being used. As we point out what the equipment is we can hold it up so that all can see.

4. We need to explain how the equipment is arranged.

5. After each step of the procedure is demonstrated, we need to stop and look at the group. Ask if they saw and understood what was done and HOW it was done. If they did not, we repeat the step before we move on to the next one.

6. We move on in this way until the entire procedure has been shown.

7. Let all the students see and touch the equipment, put it together or take it apart.

8. Ask one of the students to repeat the demonstration. Encourage the student by remarks like "that's good", "that's fine".

9. Each one should be given the same chance to practise, even if the students have to work among themselves in the afternoon and evening.

Each skill, like each problem, is different. But some conditions are common to all, such as:-

- before giving any equipment we must know exactly what is to be done with it

- we must prepare the equipment we need and put it together

- if necessary it must be sterilized (e.g. scissors, syringes)

- we must prepare the solutions and drugs we need

- before beginning, we must explain to the patient what we are going to do and why, and what result we expect.

(i) Giving an Injection

Let us take an example of how to learn a manual skill, such as "how to give an injection". We need to relate it to a problem, e.g. Problem 4.2 in the Working Guide.

We could illustrate the problem by story-telling or acting. Let us say a young boy falls from a tree and cuts his leg. We need to see where the wound is, if it is bleeding ... (follow the questions in the Working Guide).

Following the Working Guide you may compose a story where you outline the steps to take when you first see the little boy. Use the steps in the Working Guide to build up the end of your story.

You will see when you study the problem (and as suggested in the Working Guide) that if the wound is big and dirty you may have to give an injection of penicillin every day for three days.

How do we learn to give an injection? It is most important that we do not harm the patient. It must cause the least possible risk and the least possible pain. Ask the group if they have ever had an injection. If so, where did the needle go? did it hurt? etc. In this way you lead the group to think about the feelings and fears of the patient.

At the same time the group must understand that it is not the injection itself that cures, which is what many people believe, but the drug which is injected.

Many people believe that injections are a quick cure and have faith in them. We need to learn, and get patients, and especially mothers of young children, to understand that some very good drugs are taken by mouth and not injected at all.

Why are injections given? By questions and answers students will learn the following:

Reasons for giving drugs by injection

(a) If they were taken by mouth, some drugs would be made weak or destroyed by fluid (juices) in the stomach

(b) Some injected drugs act for a long time in the body; e.g. procaine penicillin - one injection a day is enough

(c) Usually medicines act more quickly by injection than by mouth

(d) Injections are always used when a patient is not able to take a drug by mouth because he is vomiting or is unconscious.

STEP I: How to explain to the patient and/or family what you (PHW) are going to do

The PHW must recognize that this first step is very important. Suggest that one PHW acts the role of the patient and another acts the role of the PHW, who will explain what he is going to do, why he is doing it, and where he will put the needle. We should remember that small children are especially afraid of injections and have to be handled gently. The PHW can learn in the dispensary how to instruct a mother to hold a child.

- 312 -

<u>STEP II</u>: How to prepare the equipment and material

Remember the importance of <u>cleanliness</u>: the PHW must have clean hands
and clean, short finger-nails. The equipment must be clean and the patient
must be clean. Why? Here you can link up learning to other problems where
the same technique and principles apply, e.g. Problem 4.1 "Burns" includes
cleaning the skin, hand-washing, etc. Let each PHW look at the drawing in the
Working Guide and select what is needed for an injection. In this way they will
learn to identify and handle the equipment. They can practise taking care of
equipment, how to clean it, how to put a syringe together, how to hold it, how
to handle it for an injection.

<u>STEP III</u>: How to give an injection (this is additional to pages 254-258 of
the Working Guide)

The angle at which the needle is inserted is important. It is shown here:

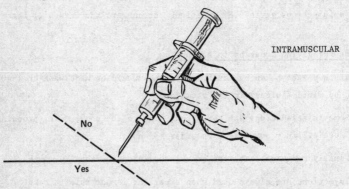

INTRAMUSCULAR

No

Yes

<u>The needle must be sharp</u>. Before boiling the needle, check that it is sharp
by running a finger along the tip and passing the needle through cotton wool. A
sharp needle should not pick up any wool. Sharpen a needle by rubbing it on a very
smooth stone.

<u>The needle and syringe must be sterile</u>.
Wrap the syringe and needle in a clean cloth
and <u>BOIL</u> for ten minutes.

When giving many injections at one time you
may not be able to boil the needles. You can
pass a needle through the flame of a spirit
lamp for just long enough for a spitting sound
to be heard. Do not heat it so much that it
becomes red. If you have a thumb forceps use
it to pick up the boiled needles, or wash your
hands first. <u>NEVER LET ANYTHING</u> (flies, fingers,
clothes) <u>TOUCH A BOILED OR FLAMED NEEDLE.</u>

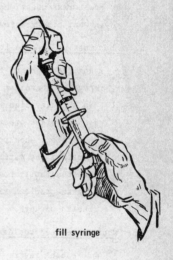

attach needle

   <u>Place the patient as needed according to what</u>
<u>part of the body will receive the injection.</u>
Children are afraid of injections. Hold them
well when you give the injection.

   <u>Clean the skin of the injection with a soapy</u>
<u>sponge.</u>

   <u>Draw up the drug into the sterile syringe.</u>
See the drawing.

   <u>Keep the needle sterile before and after you have</u>
<u>drawn the drug into the syringe.</u> If you have to put
the syringe down, lay it on a raised surface so that
the needle does not touch anything.

   <u>Inject the drug into the patient.</u>

fill syringe

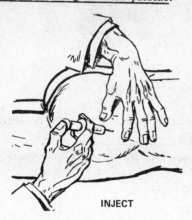

INJECT

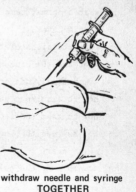

withdraw needle and syringe
TOGETHER

   To teach the intramuscular injection in the buttock, and the subcutaneous
injection, follow the steps outlined in the Working Guide, pages 254 to 258.

(ii) Taking the Temperature and Examining the Patient

Other examples of manual skills are taking the temperature and examining a patient. Read Problem 1.2 in the Working Guide, "Fever". Following the method used to learn other problems let us break down the problem of fever.

1. What do we need to know?

    - what FEVER is (see page 11, Problem 1.2)
    - what shows that fever is present
    - how it occurs
    - how to prevent fever
    - how to ask questions and find out the possible causes of fever
    - in what diseases fever is a danger sign (e.g. malaria).

2. What must we be able to do? We must be able to:

    - recognize signs of fever
    - recognize the other signs of the most common diseases of which fever
        is a danger sign
    - give the right treatment for fever, according to the signs present
    - take action, when possible, to prevent fever
    - understand the markings on the temperature chart
    - teach the family how to care for a patient with fever
    - recognize serious signs and when to refer a patient to other
        health workers.

3. What do we need to learn?

    - what causes fever
    - what a normal temperature is
    - what a fever is
    - what the signs of fever are
    - what are the diseases that are accompanied by fever and are
        especially dangerous in your area
    - how to examine a patient with fever (see point 1.2.2 under Problem 1.2)
    - how to take the temperature
    - how to read the thermometer (see page 252) and write the temperature on
        the chart
    - how to take the pulse and count the breathing

- how to clean the thermometer and prevent it from being broken
- how to know which problem to refer to in the Working Guide when fever
  is present
- how to give the right treatment - by mouth or by injection
- how to give fluids
- how to make a patient comfortable and to advise the family concerning
  care and when to return to see the PHW.

STEP I

A combination of methods is used. The causes of fever can be discussed in
a group. Students can begin by asking each other: "Have you ever had a fever?
What kind of fever (local name)? How did it begin? What did you or your mother
do about it? What kind of treatment did you have? Did you get well quickly?"
Then ask how the people in your community usually treat fever. One student could
write the answers on the blackboard. Building on this, the group will come to
understand what causes fever. When a person has a fever it is a sign that the
body is sick. Germs, which we cannot see, enter the body. They begin to multiply.
The body tries to fight the germs and kill them. Sometimes the body is not strong
enough and the person becomes ill. Fever is a sign that a fight is going on in
the body. But treatment (medicine by mouth or by injection) may be needed also
to help the body to kill the germs and get well again.

Discuss the treatment given locally. Emphasize its good points, e.g. giving
a feverish person plenty to drink. If, however, certain practices appear to be
harmful, such as not giving a feverish person anything to drink, this should be
discussed to learn why it is harmful and why it should be discouraged.

STEP II: Practice

Next, examine a patient and take the temperature; we must learn the correct
procedures. The students can take one another's temperature, read the thermometers,
practise writing the temperature on the chart and reading a temperature chart. The
same method can be used to learn why and how we take the pulse and count the
respirations (breaths). Then students must practise these skills in the dispensary
or in patients' homes. They also learn to watch patients, how they look and behave.
Do they look tired? Do they seem to be in pain? What other signs are present?
Remember that fever is only one sign of sickness; there may be other signs.

We have to remember that in a health centre or dispensary many people may be waiting for treatment, and the health worker may not have much time for teaching; so we have to watch carefully how he does his work, before we can do these things ourselves.

We learn first by watching or observing. Then we learn by <u>examining</u> patients, using our hands gently to find out what is not normal; e.g. the skin is very hot, the patient feels pain when we press a certain part of the body.

At the same time, the skills we have learned about <u>talking with people</u> will be used. But we must remember the patient is ill - ask only the most important questions such as: were you well yesterday? did you eat or drink? do you feel more ill today? where is the pain? etc. Try to reassure the patient so that he will not be too worried.

<u>STEP III</u>: Writing down results

PHWs should write down what they observe and the results of the examinations so that they can be discussed with the other health workers and later among themselves. This will lead to discussion of treatment. Discuss signs again, look for the corresponding problem in the Working Guide. Note the treatment you must give. If the medicine is to be given by injection, see the section on how to give an injection (pages 254-258).

<u>STEP IV</u>: Helping the patient to get well and keep well

When the sickness is over, talk with the patient and explain the causes of the sickness. Talk about how to keep well, how to prevent the sickness from coming back, how to prevent it from going to other people.

Using a combination of methods

We have already discussed a variety of teaching methods that we can use according to the problem we are dealing with. We have also referred to a combination of methods, and shown how different methods can be used such as story-telling, play-acting and manual skills. To understand the use of a combination of methods we shall now discuss another example.

This deals with a common and quite normal event, which may, however, become a problem if we are not careful and do not do certain things.

The example is the birth of a child, which begins when the mother becomes pregnant and continues after the baby is born.

If we refer to the Working Guide it will include Problems 2.1, 2.2, 2.3, 2.4 and 3.1.

Breaking the problem down

A.   <u>What do we need to know?</u> first:

A.1 Is the woman pregnant? If we look at the first page of Problem 2.1 (page 43), we find a brief description of the signs of pregnancy. We may add to this description that, as the months go by, other signs will appear: the breasts become bigger, later the nipple becomes darker and fluid may come out of the breast. The expectant mother may want to pass urine frequently, and the baby moves and kicks.

A.2 The woman is pregnant. We must understand what happens to a woman normally from the beginning when the baby is first formed inside (this is called <u>conception</u>) to the end, when the baby comes out (this is <u>delivery</u> or <u>childbirth</u>). We must know how to maintain a healthy pregnancy:

> what to eat
>
> rest and movement
>
> passing stools and urine
>
> when to visit the PHW or village midwife.

A.3 Recognize when something is wrong.

(a)   early signs such as:

> vomiting
>
> bleeding
>
> tiredness
>
> abdominal pain
>
> swelling of feet
>
> other illnesses (cold, cough, fever ...)

and what to do if such signs appear.

(b) dangerous signs (usually appear in the later months of pregnancy, after five months):

> continuous vomiting
>
> heavy bleeding
>
> fainting
>
> headaches
>
> swelling of feet, hands and perhaps face
>
> severe abdominal pain or abdomen is hard and large
>
> baby does not move
>
> other illnesses (cough, fever, diarrhoea, etc.)

B.   In order to obtain the information we need we should be able to:

B.1 Talk with a woman, ask questions and listen.

B.2 Write down certain things such as:

> age of woman, number of children she already has, date of last menstruation (period), general health.

B.3 Examine the woman. Is she healthy? Examine the abdomen; how many months has she been pregnant? Weigh her. Ask her questions and listen to her complaints, if any. When possible, test her urine, take her blood-pressure, take her temperature and pulse (follow techniques in the Working Guide).

B.4 Advise and teach the expectant mother what to do. Explain to her:

- how to keep well, what to eat and drink
- which signs to look for to see if something is wrong; where to go for help or advice; when to visit you
- how to prepare for the birth of the baby
- how to know when labour will start
- how to keep herself and her baby well
- breast-feeding
- birth spacing or family planning.

(See Problem 2.4 in the Working Guide).

C.   We need to learn:

- how to know when a woman is pregnant
- how to ask questions and what questions to ask; how to listen for answers
- how to write down answers in a few words

- how to examine a pregnant woman
- how to recognize signs that something is not normal
- what to do about certain signs found
- how to take the temperature, pulse and respiration
- how to test urine
- how to weigh
- how to decide which treatment to give (if any)
- when to refer (i.e. when to send the woman to see someone else, such as the nurse, midwife or doctor)
- how to teach and advise mothers how to keep up their health and the health of the family, and to prevent complications
- how to teach that breast-feeding is good
- how to teach about birth spacing or family planning (see Problem 2.4 in the Working Guide).

The methods of teaching topics A, B and C could be:

Topic A - Small-group discussion with student assignments

Topic B - Small-group discussion with story-telling and play-acting

Topic C - Learning manual skills by demonstration to groups, followed by students repeating the demonstration, and individual practice. Students can practise these skills on each other - e.g. taking each other's temperature, weight, pulse, etc.

Then we can go to Problem 2.2

The end of pregnancy: the mother will soon deliver her baby. Like pregnancy, delivery is a normal process and will usually stay normal if certain simple measures are taken. These measures will protect the mother and the child during delivery and afterwards.

Breaking the problem down

A. What do we need to know?

1. Is the woman in labour?
2. Was the pregnancy normal? If yes, one can expect a normal labour.
3. Is the bladder full, or what are the signs of a full bladder?
4. Has she passed stools today?
5. When did she last drink and eat?
6. Did she have local medicine?

7. The progress of labour: beginning, pain, kind of pain, how often the pain comes, when the baby is about to be born, signs:
   - when the baby is coming out
   - when the abdomen is hard again

8. Amount of blood: how much bleeding? A lot or a little bleeding, when bleeding must stop.

9. Condition of normal new-born baby
   - how to help its breathing.

B. What do we need to do

1. Examine the woman to see if labour has begun (note Point 1 on page 58 in Working Guide)[1]

2. Prepare mother for labour (refer to Point 2). Prepare the place where the birth will be, e.g. a clean bed or mat, boiled water, clean clothes, clean baby clothes.

3. Deliver the baby (follow Point 3 on page 60).

4. Take care of the baby immediately after birth.

5. Deliver the afterbirth and examine it (follow Point 4 on page 62).

6. Take care of the mother.

C. What do we need to learn

1. The signs of labour, normal and abnormal.

2. How to use what we know about the pregnancy.

3. To recognize when labour pains become stronger.

4. How to encourage a woman to pass urine.

5. How to give an enema if no stools were passed today.

6. Signs that the baby is about to be born.

7. What the bag of waters is, how it protects the baby's head, and what happens when the bag of water breaks.

8. What to do to prepare for the delivery of the baby (see Point 2 on page 58 in the Working Guide).

9. How to deliver the baby.

10. What to do if the delivery is not normal; e.g. the buttocks or the feet come out first, or the shoulder comes out first, or the cord is twisted around the neck.

---

[1] Be sure to encourage her to pass urine. This can be done, for example, by pouring warm water over the genitals while she squats. Also see that she has passed stools; if NOT, give her an enema.

11. After the baby is born:
     - how to wrap the baby
     - how to clear the baby's mouth and nose of fluid
     - how to cut and treat the cord (local customs must be considered)
     - how to put eyedrops in the baby's eyes.

12. How to know when the afterbirth is ready to come out - what to do; how
     to know when the bleeding is too much and what to do (e.g. rubbing
     up a contraction by massaging the abdomen; see Point 4.7 on page 63);
     what to do if the afterbirth has not come out.

13. How to take care of the mother.

14. How to clean the mother and make her comfortable.

15. How to wash the new-born baby and weigh it, and look for signs that are
     not normal.

16. How to clean and tidy up the equipment.

17. After the mother has rested, how and _when_ to talk with her about taking
     care of her new-born baby. When to come again to visit the PHW for
     check-up and further advice, or when the PHW will visit her at home.
     The PHW will also advise her when the first vaccination (BCG, for
     instance) can be done.

18. How and what to teach the family about the mother's diet (what to eat),
     the importance of fluids, and how to take care of her during the next
     few days, especially watch for:
     - bleeding
     - fever
     - cramps
     - bad-smelling discharge
     and if any of these occur to immediately inform the PHW.

19. What to do if the mother has fever, bleeding, cramps, bad-smelling
     discharge.

20. How to advise the mother or another family member how to take care of
     the baby, especially the _cord_, and to call the PHW if there is any
     discharge from the _cord_ or from the baby's eyes, or if any red spots
     appear on the skin.

21. How to take care of the child (see Problem 3.1, "Feeding the child").

22. How to use and fill in the growth chart.

23. How to write the record card.

24. How and _when_ to immunize children.

25. How to advise parents on birth spacing or family planning so that
    mothers may regain their strength and keep up their health.

26. Where to send mothers or fathers for help with birth spacing or
    family planning.

Methods to use for Problem 2.2

To learn about care during and after labour, for the mother and baby, again we
can use a combination of methods. Section A, about what we need to know, can be
taught in group discussions; we can use drawings or models of a woman's pelvis and
a baby inside. This can be used to show how the baby moves down and comes out of the
mother. To learn about contractions we can use a balloon which can be filled with air
at intervals and covered with a cushion to muffle the sound. This will help to give
a feeling of the abdomen becoming hard with pain and soft when the pain goes away.
These are a combination of the methods of group discussion and demonstration, students
repeating the demonstration and practising the process themselves.

After everyone understands the process, it can be followed up by, first,
observation of a delivery in the maternity hospital or at home. This would be followed
by individual practice in order to gain skill and confidence. At this point there must
be one teacher with one student; the student delivers the baby with the teacher's help
(the teacher at this point may well be a staff member of the local maternity hospital
or clinic). Two other students could observe and help during the delivery. Manual
skills and observation skills must also be learned for the various procedures, e.g.
how to deliver the baby and the placenta, how to clean the cord, how to clean the
eyes, how to immunize a baby, how to record events, how to prepare and maintain
equipment, etc.

Once we know how to deal with Problems 2.1, 2.2, 2.3, 2.4 and 3.1 in the Working
Guide, we can then approach the community and do the following:

1. Find out where the pregnant women are, and how many there are, in
   the village we serve (read "Approaching the community", page 290).

2. Find out how many children there are under five (read "Approaching the
   community", page 290).

3. Organize a meeting with groups of mothers to talk about mother and
   child care; after the meeting, arrange to meet each woman individually
   at her home to discuss what to do in pregnancy and how to take care of

herself and her family. The mothers and the PHW should decide
together when they should see each other again.

4.   Talk with mothers about when to immunize their children and who will
     do it; when to discuss how to keep themselves in good health, e.g.
       - nutrition
       - birth spacing or family planning.

5.   Organize meetings for the discussion and demonstration of food and
     nutrition matters and the prevention of illness.

6.   Other subjects that are raised during the meeting should be discussed
     later with the women.

TALKING WITH PEOPLE ABOUT HEALTH

A sick person can often be cured of his sickness. But while he is sick he
loses time from work (or from learning at school); and some sicknesses, even when
they are cured, leave the person weak and easily tired for a long time afterwards.
So, although it may be much easier to show that we have helped to cure a person,
it is much more important, and better for the person, if we can prevent the sickness.

How can we do this?

Most of the things that can be done to prevent sickness have to be done by
the person himself (in the case of babies and young children by the mother or other
person who looks after them) and sometimes by the community working together. So
our task must be to help people to understand the causes of sickness and how to
prevent it. It is equally important to help people to stay healthy and to show
them how to become stronger. We must talk to people, perhaps show them how to do
certain things, and show them pictures.

When do we talk to people?

People who are very sick, or whose children are very sick, will not want to
listen to anything except how to cure the sickness. But when they are getting
better they may be prepared to talk and to listen about how to prevent sickness.

If there is much sickness (an epidemic) in the village those who are not yet
sick may be willing to think about ways to stop the sickness: e.g. prevention may
mean safeguarding the water supply, and, although it cannot be done at once, people
may be willing to discuss it and agree to do something when the epidemic has finished,
or when planting or harvesting is over.

Sometimes, quite unexpectedly, people who are well will ask a question which gives us a chance to talk about prevention. Even though nothing may happen at once, the person may go and think about what has been discussed. Later he may ask more questions or talk to others, and they will ask questions. It may take a long time, and many explanations, but at last something may change if we do not try to make people act too quickly.

Whom do we talk to?

We may talk to individual people, to groups, or to the whole village. People must do some things for themselves, but it is easier to change what we are doing if a number of people agree together to make the change and to help one another. So, very often we may need to talk with people by themselves, but also with small groups such as mothers of young babies, so that they can discuss the new ways and agree on what to do.

If the whole village must decide on something, for example, to protect the water supply so that it does not bring sickness, then we must ask the chief or responsible person to call a village meeting. It will be easier at the village meeting if we have already talked with some individual people, and explained what is needed and why, so that they already understand and will help to explain things to others. It is especially important for the village leaders and influential people to understand the problem before the meeting begins.

What about customs and taboos?

Often how people behave and what they do are things which have always been done that way by the people. The old teach the young, and everyone behaves in the same way. Some of these old ways are good. We should try to find such good ways and help the older people to teach others to keep these ways. This should please them, and make them more ready to listen if we want to talk about changing other ways.

Some of the old ways may not be very good, but if they do no harm, there is no need to try to change them. They are not important enough for us to change them, so we can forget about them.

Some old customs, however, are not good. We should look carefully at these. These old ways, for example, often tell us that good food must be kept for the men and not given to women or young children. We should talk quietly with the elders to find out why these old ways are kept. Perhaps they were once important (when men had to fight to protect their families, for example) but they may not be quite so important now. Try to get the elders to think about these old ways, and maybe after a while they will agree to help you to change them. This is very important, but if they refuse to change, do not openly and directly oppose them. Try to make people think a little about the problem, and be patient. If the elders oppose you, you will find it very difficult or even impossible to work in the village. In time, and with the help of others such as the teacher, the agricultural extension worker and others, the elders may see the need for change; or there will be enough people in the village who agree together so that they will quietly make the change.

How do we talk with people?

The first and best way is to know how to listen to others when we ask such questions as: What do you think about health? What do you think about this idea? Can you propose new things that will help yourselves or others? Do you understand what I am proposing? <u>Listen first</u>, and most of the time; then you can talk.

There are many ways of bringing new ideas to people. We may talk directly. We may answer questions. We may ask questions and leave people to think or talk about the answers. We may help people to make up songs, or dances, or plays or stories. We may ask story-tellers or players to do so. We may ask others (supervisor, other workers, visitors) to talk to people. We may show pictures - flannelgraphs, photographs, flip-charts, etc. We may use the visit of a film show. We may get people to listen together to a radio broadcast.

Whichever way we use, it is the people themselves who must decide to make a change. We cannot force them. We can only go on explaining, answering questions, helping them to think things out for themselves. We ourselves, of course, must always behave the way we wish others to behave. Our example may often be the best way of finally persuading others.

3.

Evaluation

1. <u>HOW CAN WE KNOW THE PURPOSES OF TRAINING HAVE BEEN ATTAINED?</u>

To evaluate is to seek to understand what we are doing and perhaps why we are not achieving what we hoped to achieve. We have referred to evaluation often in this book, e.g. when we asked the student to demonstrate certain skills, by questioning and talking with students about a story to find out if the message we wanted to give had been understood. Evaluation is an essential part of training as it is of almost everything we do in life:

- we know when rice is cooked and is tender and good to eat. If
  we do not cook it long enough it is hard and not good to eat
- we know how much time we need to go to the market, etc.

<u>If we think of the student</u>, evaluation is necessary to help him to see:

- how well he is learning what he should be learning
- why he is not doing better
- in what respects he is strong or weak
- how he can be helped to improve.

It can encourage the student who is doing well to continue learning.

The student himself should take part in the evaluation. He must know the result of the evaluation so that he knows the weaknesses and strengths of the particular learning activity and <u>build on the strengths</u>. This is to help him and not to punish him.

If we think of the teacher, evaluation is the best way for him to know the result of his work. The teacher helps the student by reacting to the student's effort to learn. Often students do not learn because the teacher is not a good and encouraging teacher.

If we think of the training programme, evaluation helps to find out whether the objectives of the training programme have been achieved, i.e. if the student can do what the programme was designed to train him to do. It also indicates where and how the programme may be improved. For example, we may find that what the student has learned about infant feeding cannot be applied usefully when he teaches mothers in the village because, perhaps, people do not believe in giving certain food to children. We should then find out the taboos behind this belief and then give a bigger place in the programme to finding out about taboos and customs.

2. WHEN SHOULD WE EVALUATE?

Evaluation goes on all the time. It starts with the learning objectives, which themselves may need to be revised, and from there it continues as shown in the teaching module. It is used while students learn about the different problems to see how they are progressing, and where they need further help or individual attention. Later, when they work in the community, evaluation is used to find out whether what they learned is useful, or if there are problems for which they were not properly trained.

Another way that evaluation can show that training was good is to see the PHWs working with interest and satisfaction, staying in their work, increasing it, and seeing that the community is satisfied with the services they give.

All this information is used to improve the learning and teaching programme.

3. HOW CAN EVALUATION BE DONE?

During learning and teaching activities many opportunities arise for evaluation. The training of PHWs is concerned mainly with the students' ability to do certain things, to perform practical tasks.

Some types of evaluation that can be used are:

- <u>The teacher can observe, and students and the teacher can ask questions</u>,
  during practical work, story-telling, play-acting and home-visiting.
  This will show if the student is progressing and learning more.

- <u>The teacher talking with (not to) the student</u> has the advantage of personal
  contact which helps to find out what the student really knows, feels, etc.

- <u>Group discussion</u> during which the teacher will observe the student's
  participation, especially his contribution to discussion, and how he
  says and judges what to do in certain situations.

- <u>Observation</u> is not only looking. It is also finding out - e.g. such
  information as the following:

    - how did the student try to find out about a problem?
    - what action did he take?
    - did he choose the right moment to teach an individual or a group,
      and did he use the proper words?
    - did he give a demonstration?
    - did he listen properly and encourage the group to ask questions?
    - did he give the right answer?

- <u>Questioning</u> is another way of evaluating what the student knows; this
  means that the teacher should listen carefully and patiently. The
  following are some examples of questioning:

    - At the end of a day the teacher could ask the student:

        What was the most interesting thing you did today?
        Why?
        Did you discover anything new?

    <u>OR</u>

    - At the end of the visit to the community the teacher could ask
      the students:

        What did you see?
        What did you do?
        How did you feel about it?

4. <u>WHAT ARE THE ASPECTS WITH WHICH THE TEACHER SHOULD BE CONCERNED WHEN
   EVALUATING LEARNING AND TEACHING</u>

Three things are important for the teacher to remember when evaluating
learning:

   (i)   If the teacher wants to find out how much the student knows and can
         do about, e.g. burns, he must ask the student those questions and
         observe those actions that are related to burns. Questions about fever
         in this case would not be as important as questions about infection.

   (ii) If the teacher wants to find out if his questions are good he should
         obtain almost the same answer from each student in the group to the
         same questions.

   (iii) If the teacher wants to avoid making a wrong judgement about a
         learning experience, he can prepare in advance the most important
         answers to particular questions, as shown in the following example:

Questions	Answers
Say when any medicine can be a poison	- if it is given to the wrong person - if the wrong amount is given
Say when a medicine is useless	- if it is not taken by the patient - if it is not taken at the right time - if it is not taken long enough
When you give medicine say what you must make sure your patients understand	- how much medicine they should take - how often they should take it - how long they should take it for

5. <u>WHAT TO DO WITH THE RESULTS OF EVALUATION</u>

When evaluating a student the following may be found, as shown in the drawing:

1) he knows but cannot do

2) he does not know but he can do

3) he knows and can do

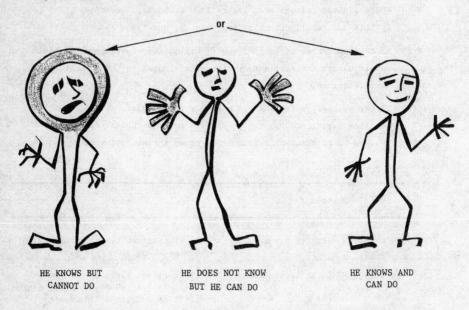

| HE KNOWS BUT CANNOT DO | HE DOES NOT KNOW BUT HE CAN DO | HE KNOWS AND CAN DO |

OUTCOME OF LEARNING

The learning process is aimed at producing a person who knows the important things about his task and can perform that task. Therefore, we must compare the results of evaluation with the learning objectives to see if he has learned all he should have learned. If he has not, we can help him to correct the weak points. For example, <u>a student who does not know all he should</u> about a task but can perform the task, such as "can very well weigh a baby but does not understand the danger of the baby becoming thinner or how to teach the mother to give her baby the right food", must spend more time learning to understand this danger and practising this teaching.

<u>For one who knows about a task and can answer questions and teach others well</u>
but is not able correctly to carry out important tasks like applying a dressing or
giving an injection, we must help him to correct what is wrong and to spend more time
at practical work. So we see why it is important to write down what the student
should be able to do at the end of his training (learning objectives); you can then
see if he has learned these skills (evaluation) and when and why to go back to correct
what is wrong and continue to develop what is good.

4.

Examples

of

learning modules

A "learning module" is a planned set of activities
which will assist the student (the PHW) to
develop a specified competence.

Learning modules can be elaborated for each problem presented in the Working Guide (Part I). They can facilitate both learning and teaching by organizing them in a logical way.

Following are two examples of learning modules designed around two problems in the Working Guide, namely:

1. "The badly-fed child" (Problem 3.2, page 93)

2. "Burns" (Problem 4.1, page 99)

The sequence is the following:

1. The problem is stated;

2. Learning objectives are defined;

3. The teacher finds out what the PHWs already know about the problem;

4. The learning content, as in the Working Guide, is then divided into what the PHW should know (knowledge) and what he should do (skills);

5. What a PHW has already learned is referred to and used;

6. Learning and teaching methods are selected, listed and used in order of importance; and

7. The progress made by the PHW is assessed.

The same process can be used for each of the thirty-four problems dealt with in Part I, as well as for those which will be identified and studied to meet the needs of a given community. Teacher-training centres, and WHO or other advisers can assist you in this task, if necessary.

Example 1: "The badly-fed child" (see Part I, Problem 3.2)

Learning objectives	Finding out what the PHW already knows about this problem	Content (from the Working Guide)		Using what a PHW has already learned	Learning/teaching methods*	How is the PHW progressing (Evaluation)
		What a PHW must know	What a PHW must do			
To be able to: -weigh a child -decide whether the child has the right weight for his age -recognize 3 major signs of malnutrition -show a mother how to prepare a bottle of liquid to feed a child suffering from malnutrition -tell in what cases a PHW would send a child suffering from severe malnutrition to the hospital or health centre.	Has he seen a malnourished child? or heard of one? What did he look like? What was done for the child? Did he get better or worse or die?, etc.	Review briefly the growth and development of a child. Early signs of malnutrition: -persistent crying -diarrhoea -getting thinner -not growing well Severe signs of malnutrition: -skin creases (the child just skin and bone) -eyes dull -does not eat -vomits -diarrhoea -fever -swelling of legs, feet and hands -hair changes colour Treatment: -replacing lost liquid -changing or correcting child's diet Signs of improvement or getting worse When and where to refer? How to organize a community gathering for health teaching.	Examine a child Weigh a child Use weight chart Talk with mother Demonstrate how to prepare food for child and how to give it and return demonstration by the mother Give liquid mixture Give medicine Prepare and clean equipment Send sick child to hospital or health centre	-How to compare the weight of healthy child with the age of the child -How a baby grows and develops - Feeding the child -Local food customs and habits -Advantages of birth spacing for mother and child -Nutrition	●Observation of how mothers feed their children (house, dispensary, market) and talk to them ●Find out local food habits and customs, what food available (special assignment), watching and giving demonstration ●Talking with people about healthy nutrition ●Getting the help of the agricultural extension worker to teach local people to grow food ●Practise work in a dispensary, home visiting ●Group discussion (students talk about the growth and development of children, their own or others) ●Play-acting * Give each method listed here a priority number in order to begin by the ones you consider the most important and leave aside those you may not have enough time to deal with.	Ways of evaluating this: Observation of the PHW - During weighing the child: Did he check that the scale is balanced? Did he hold the child safely? Did he talk with child and/or his mother? Did he read the correct weight and write it on the chart? - How did he examine the child, e.g. did he press the skin to see if there is swelling of the leg, or if the skin creases? - How did he teach the mother about giving fluid to her child, did he show her how to do it? - Did he prepare and clean equipment? - Practising other tasks: Giving fluid or medicine, demonstrating about food with the mother at home and/or women in the community. Questioning (oral and written), and listening - Is the weight of the child correct for its age? If not, why not? - What would you do for him? - How would you know if he is improving? - How can you tell it is becoming serious? What would you do for him? - What can you do to prevent this problem? - What can the mother do? - What can the community do? And who can help? - What did you know about this problem in your special assignment?

Example 2:   "Burns"   (see Part I, Problem 4.1)

Learning objectives	Finding out what the PHW already knows about this problem	Content (from the Working Guide) — What a PHW must know	What a PHW must do	Using what a PHW has already learned	Learning/teaching methods*	How is the PHW progressing (Evaluation)
To be able to: -decide whether the burn covers a small or large area -decide when a patient with burns should be sent to the hospital or health centre -recognize whether the skin is covered with blisters only -recognize whether the skin is broken or has been removed -clean a wound -treat blisters and skin which is broken or has been removed -treat a wound that smells bad or from which a yellowish fluid is coming out -tell the patient and his family how to prevent burns	Has he or someone in his family ever been burned? What did they do for this burn? What happened to the person who was burned?	What causes burns How to prevent burns The danger of a large area of skin being burned How to keep the burn clean and prevent infection (clean hands, control of flies ...) When large area of the skin has been burned First aid, taking a temperature, giving an injection (techniques) The importance of giving fluid When small area of the skin has been burned Recognize and treat blisters Techniques of dressing What advice to give to the patient or his family How to recognize complications (fever, discharge, bad swelling) and when to refer How to organize community gathering for health teaching	Teach the prevention of burns (protect children from fire and boiling water) Give first aid Put on dressing Give fluid Take a temperature Give penicillin injection or treatment as prescribed Send patient to the hospital Follow up the patient treatment Refer in case of complication Prepare and clean equipment.	-How to do a dressing, an injection, take a temperature -How microbes spread infections (as described under "Fever") -How flies aggravate infection (as described in "Waste disposal")	● Observation of a burned person ● Practical experience in treating a burn ● Group discussion about burns (severe, mild, complications)... ● Drawing on blackboard by teachers and students ● Review demonstration of dressing techniques	Ways of evaluating this: Observation of the PHW - Are his hands clean? - How does he examine the patient? - Does he examine the patient gently? - Does he speak with the patient or his family and reassure them? - Does he give the right treatment according to whether the burn area is large or small? - Does he prepare the necessary equipment and clean it afterwards? - Practising other tasks: Taking the temperature, giving the injection, doing the dressing. Teaching the patient and the community. Questioning (oral and written) and listening - Is it serious; why? - Is he giving fluid; why? If not, why not? - Why is the patient being sent to the hospital or the health centre? - For which complications does he refer the patient - What would make you change the treatment? - How was the patient burned? - What other things cause burns? - How can you prevent burns? - How can you prevent burns in the community? - How can the community help?

* Give each method listed here a priority number in order to begin by the ones you consider the most important and leave aside those you may not have enough time to deal with.

PART III

★

Guidelines

for

adapting this book

★ ★ ★

GUIDELINES FOR ADAPTING

this book to suit national situations

———————

1. INTRODUCTION

It is impossible to write a working guide for universal application. Local
conditions vary from country to country according not only to the level of development
but also to the geographical situation and to the culture, habits and preferences.
Even within the same country there may be significant differences. It is important,
therefore, to adapt this to suit local health problems and to suit what is expected
of a country's health manpower.

Adaptation is not always an easy task. The following guidelines have been
prepared in the hope that national health administrators will find them useful when
adapting this book for the use of their own primary health workers. The adaptation
is best done locally by people well acquainted with the prevailing situation, habits
and culture.

2. PREREQUISITES

The preparation of teaching/learning material for primary health workers is
not the first step in the development of primary health care in a country. It will
usually be preceded by the commitment of the government to cover the population through
a network of primary health care services, followed by the adoption of a health policy
that guides and backs up those responsible for the preparation of the training
programmes. In some cases primary health care on a national scale develops from
a pilot scheme or schemes on a local scale to test the most suitable methods for
wider adoption.

The PHW is part of the health care delivery system. He is the end link in
the chain of health service, or to put it differently, he is the peripheral member
of the health team, which may include at the intermediate level the medical assistant
or head nurse and at the next level the first physician. Thus the PHW must not be
trained nor asked to work in isolation, and his performance should be closely followed.

The medical assistant or other responsible officer must provide guidance and support as a routine responsibility. The other echelons of the health services are there to take care of referred cases and to provide logistics and in-service training as required.

Adequate supervision and a proper referral system, as part of the primary health care scheme of a country, are prerequisites to the adaptation of this book to national conditions.

3. APPOINTMENT OF A WORKING GROUP

The Minister of Health could appoint a working group to adapt the present working guide. It should be a small group which could call for assistance on specialists or other advisers.

The group should be chosen from among health administrators, public health physicians, nurse/midwives, medical assistants in charge of rural health centres, physicians of rural hospitals, sanitarians and community development personnel.

Its terms of reference would be to follow the steps of the adaptation process indicated below.

4. ADAPTATION PROCESS

4.1 Reviewing the implications of a PHC programme

This first step is to ascertain that the prerequisite conditions for the preparation of teaching/learning material for PHWs have been met, namely, whether the country is ready to begin to train PHWs.

To begin to train PHWs before their place has been carefully planned and prepared would be wrong: left to themselves or without proper supervision and guidance, PHWs might very quickly become harmful and lose the discipline and motivation needed to perform their duties effectively.

The concept of PHW should be well understood and accepted by health personnel, community leaders and the population if their support and participation is to be obtained. No durable success can be achieved without their support and participation. They are essential for good cooperation between the three levels of the district health service - the village, where PHWs work; the health centre, in the charge usually of a medical assistant; and the district or rural hospital, where a physician usually functions as the leader of the PHC team.

4.2 Deciding upon problems to be tackled by a PHW

Several constraints will influence this decision, the first of which is the role of the health team. Since the PHW is a member of that team, what he does will depend on what the others deal with as their functions are complementary and related. For instance, while the physician at a rural hospital performs caesarean section and the medical assistant or public health nurse at a rural health centre inserts IUDs, the PHW looks after normal pregnant women and treats their minor ailments while he refers abnormal conditions to the nurse or physician. Other factors which will determine the kind of work he undertakes are his previous education, the resources available, the stage of development of the country, the quality of supervision, and the referral system.

Because of the elementary nature of his education and training, the PHW should not be overloaded. His functions may be shared by other PHWs. Thus a male PHW may undertake environmental health work and a female worker be responsible for maternal and child health work.

The following criteria have been suggested for assigning priority to problems (Introduction, page 4):

- frequency of the disease
- demand from the public
- danger to the individual
- danger to the community
- technical feasibility of action for a PHW
- economic consequences of the problem.

On these criteria the thirty-four problems identified in Part I of the present book have been selected. They are grouped under seven main headings, namely:

1. Communicable diseases
2. Maternal care
3. Child health - Nutrition
4. Accidents
5. Village and home sanitation
6. Other common problems
7. Community development.

To these could be added: "Management" including record-keeping, reporting, and referral of patients. This list could serve as a framework or starting-point for the working group to identify the problems to be tackled by a PHW.

4.3 <u>Deciding upon skills authorized for a PHW</u>

At what technical level should the PHW deal with each problem? For instance:

- What role should a PHW play in maternity care, delivery, etc.?
- Should a PHW know how to detect albumin and sugar in urine? (If so, he should be given the means to do it)
- What medicines could a PHW use or give? (See Part I, page 248)
- Should a PHW give injections? If so, which ones?
- Should a PHW be able to extract a tooth?
- Which form(s) should he regularly fill in?

4.4 <u>Reviewing the job description of the PHW</u>

The PHW's job and training will depend upon the problems he has to solve and upon his technical ability. To be sure that his training fits the tasks ("task-oriented training"), the working group will write or rewrite the PHW's job description, checking it against the list of agreed problems.

The job description will serve as a basis for defining learning objectives and elaborating learning modules (see Part II, "Examples of learning modules", pages 332 to 334). It should appear as a list of tasks and duties, as shown in the following example:

The PHW will, in the community he is serving:

1. Control COMMUNICABLE DISEASES by:

    - performing vaccinations as requested by the health services, according to his supervisor's instructions
    - identifying, treating, advising and, when necessary, referring patients with fever, diarrhoea and respiratory diseases
    - preventing the spread of epidemics and keeping his supervisor informed of the appearance of epidemic cases.

2. Provide MATERNAL CARE by:

    - identifying pregnant women in the community, advising them and
        referring abnormal cases to the health centre or the hospital
    - preparing for delivery, assisting at childbirth, giving first care
        to the mother and baby, calling for assistance or referring
        patients when necessary
    - giving postnatal care, advice and family-planning information
    - advising or treating sick women or sending them to hospital.

3. Provide CHILD CARE by caring for both well-fed and badly-fed children,
    and giving nutritional advice.

4. Give PRIMARY CARE for burns, wounds, fractures and bites, and refer the
    patients when necessary.

5. Advise and educate the community on ENVIRONMENTAL HEALTH problems,
    especially on water supply, disposal of excreta and waste, and food
    protection.

6. Deal with the FOLLOWING HEALTH PROBLEMS by identifying, treating and
    referring cases when necessary: skin diseases, eye diseases, headaches,
    belly pains, pains in the joints, intestinal worms, weakness and tiredness,
    diseases of the mouth and teeth, lumps under the skin, and mental disorders.

7. Participate in COMMUNITY DEVELOPMENT by discussing community problems with
    local leaders and suggesting ways of improving the life of the people.

8. REFER all cases and problems outside or beyond his competence.

9. REPORT regularly to his supervisor and to the village committee.

This example of a job description may serve as a starting-point for any other
description of the tasks and duties a community may wish to entrust to a PHW.
Deletions and additions of problems will permit the PHW's job description to be
tailored to the priority needs of the population and of the health services. The
new job description should be included among the first pages of the national working
guide.

4.5 Identifying in the WHO working guide what problems are to be deleted
       or added

The working group will compare the job description it has drawn up (or rewritten)
with the above example from the present WHO working guide. It will thus be easy to

identify among the thirty-four problems in this book those which could be deleted
or added. A new list of problems will be established comprising both the problems
selected from this WHO working guide and those added. The former will need to be
adapted to local conditions, and the latter will have to be presented and detailed
in the same way as the former.

4.6 Adapting the problems selected from the WHO working guide

Each problem detailed in this working guide and which is included in the
rewritten job description of the PHW, must be adapted to local conditions.

The name given to the problem in the WHO guide may not be the most suitable.
For instance, Problem 2.4, "Family welfare", which deals mainly with family planning,
may need to be reworded. Some may prefer "Family planning", others "Birth spacing".
The same may apply to other problems.

The text itself has to be reviewed and adapted so that the PHW can easily
understand it. It should correspond to local habits and beliefs and regulations
of the Ministry of Health. To take the same Problem 2.4, "Family welfare", the text
should reflect national policy on family planning, and tell the PHW which contraceptives
he can recommend. Other problems will need to be similarly adapted. Certain foods are
easier to get in some countries than in others; consequently, they should be mentioned
first in the text for problems on nutrition in those countries. The text would describe
how to make the best use of the common foods and how to supplement them when necessary
by other foodstuffs the people can easily afford.

Part I, Annex 1, of the WHO working guide lists and recommends seventeen different
medicines under common names, but national health authorities may prefer other names
better known to their health workers and the public. Dosage and packaging may vary
from one country to another: they should therefore be carefully revised and modified
when necessary. Other medicines may be added, especially when they are known to be
effective and are safe, cheap and widely used. However, they should be selected very
carefully to avoid misuse, abuse and unnecessary expense.

Attention should be paid also to the drawings to be included in the adapted
working guide. For instance, pigs should not appear in countries where their meat is
not eaten. Injection techniques should not be illustrated in countries where the PHW
is not allowed to give injections. Drawings that better reflect national characteristics
and the national scene will be preferable to those in the WHO working guide.

In many countries there are official regulations and instructions with which health workers must comply; when applicable, they should be included - after revision if needed - in the national document.

4.7 Presenting and detailing the new problems added

New problems that may be added should be presented in the national document in the same way as those taken from the WHO working guide. To detail, for example, a clinical problem, one can imagine oneself in the position of a PHW who is intelligent, motivated and full of good-will, but with limited education and training. Faced with the problem, the PHW seeks advice and assistance. He must find in his working guide directives to follow and an indication of the effective and safe action he is expected to take. Each problem can be outlined in a flow-chart as indicated below in the case of Problem 4.3 "Fractures":

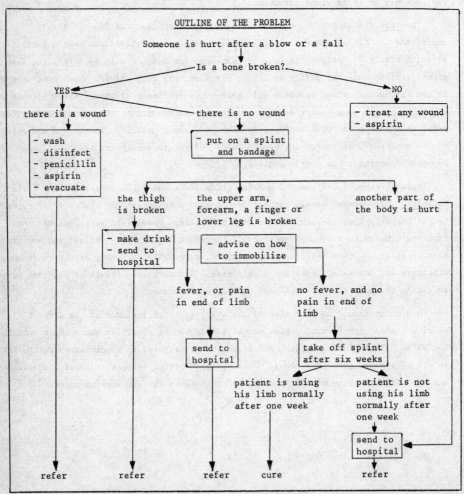

OUTLINE OF THE PROBLEM

Thus, when the PHW suspects a fracture, he can find guidance in his book, remember what he has learned and be satisfied that he has taken the right decisions. The same process can be applied to any other problem.

It may not seem advisable to include in the working guide such detailed diagrams, which are often complicated, of the various problems. However, the details they contain have proved useful in indicating the action required in a logical and simple manner.

The text should be reduced to a minimum; it should give prominence to preventive measures and official regulations and instructions. It should be illustrated by simple drawings which any PHW can easily understand. A local artist could be asked to help with illustrations.

Care should be taken to use the list of medicines already agreed upon, and any new product that is needed should be added to the list in Annex 1 of the working guide.

When dealing with management problems such as record-keeping, the supply of drugs and contraceptives, reporting, referral, supervision, and others, the instructions to the PHW should be elementary.

For record-keeping, two books could be provided to the PHW: one in which he will record his daily activities: visits, consultations and other activities, with a record of the patients and their illnesses, and births and deaths; another in which he will record drugs, contraceptives and other supplies, with the amounts received, distributed and remaining.

For reporting and referral very simple forms could be prepared so that PHWs can communicate easily among themselves and with the other levels of the health service.

Recording and reporting regulations will vary from country to country depending on the kind and amount of information a PHW will be expected to and able to provide. Similarly, the format of the forms, their number, the frequency of reporting, etc. will vary very much with local conditions.

4.8 Incorporating a simple evaluation mechanism

The objectives of the working guide are essentially twofold:

- To provide learning/teaching material during the early training of the PHW
- To serve as a reference book for practising PHWs.

To ensure that the national working guide, which will have cost much effort, has achieved its objectives it will have to be evaluated. For this, the working group will test it during a period of four to six months in the field, at two or three places with different geographical, ethnic and economic conditions. Observations will be made during and after training, and users' comments will be collected by means of a previously prepared questionnaire, asking:

- how useful the working guide has been
- where it has failed
- what difficulties have been experienced in its use
- what corrections or modifications are required
- what additions or deletions are required
- for any other comments on the content, presentation, drawings, etc.

When collected and analysed, these comments and suggestions will permit an improved new edition of the working guide; this process regularly repeated should lead in a few years to a working guide well adapted to local conditions, serving as a valuable tool for PHWs.

5. USE, TRANSLATION, PRINTING

5.1 The reason for adapting the WHO working guide to national conditions is to permit its use in national primary health care services. It can be used in two ways: as material for training and as a reference book.

When used for training, the working guide is intended mainly for PHWs. They will find listed in it a number of common and potentially dangerous problems selected by national health authorities and which a PHW can help to solve. On the first page of each problem a simple explanation is given. For instance, "pregnancy", "intestinal worms", "venereal diseases" are all technical terms the meaning of which is obvious to an educated health worker but, most probably, not to a PHW at the beginning of training.

Next, a page is devoted to learning objectives, for the benefit of both the PHW and his trainer. Stated as tasks they indicate what a PHW can do at the end of training that he could not do before. These objectives can be defined only after a job-description of the PHW has been prepared, listing those tasks. They should enable the PHW student to better understand his learning activities and why he needs to be trained.

Then follow a few pages of text, illustrated by simple drawings, which
describe how the problem can be prevented or dealt with, and the procedures
the PHW should follow. Thus, for "respiratory disease" (Problem 1.4), the
PHW is instructed to ask "for how long have you been coughing and spitting?";
the procedures he should follow will depend upon the answer - e.g. for a few
days or for weeks or months.

In his daily work the PHW will have to use the few medicines or drugs put at
his disposal, take temperatures, apply bandages and possibly give certain injections.
Indications to this effect appear in the annexes to the working guide, which will
be expanded and supplemented, as required, by the national health authorities.

Although the guide is intended primarily for PHWs, it is also essential
that all those who share responsibility in the training (physicians, medical
assistants, nurses, sanitarians, administrators) be familiar with its contents:
job-description of the PHW, learning objectives corresponding to each problem,
and annexes. One annex shows "anatomical diagrams"; it is intended mainly for
the PHWs' trainers. Some of these diagrams may be too complex and difficult for
PHWs while others may be inappropriate; this will vary from country to country.
In any case they require explanations. They can nevertheless be useful to trainers
and serve as models for their blackboard drawings.

The PHWs should keep their working guide very carefully as it will be a precious
companion to which they can refer to check the action they should take or the dose
of a medicine, or to comply with instructions and regulations. The content of the
working guide represents only a basic training which must be built on and continuously
improved. PHWs should be asked to write in it the results of their experiences, the
advice of their supervisors, and additional information they receive from the health
services.

5.2 The working document will be fully adapted only when it is translated into
local languages for use by auxiliary health personnel in rural or suburban communities.
Its translation is essential. This is a difficult and delicate task that should not
be left to any but the most skilled translator. The translation should be revised
by health technicians fully aware of local pathology; of health and medical terminology;

and of local usages, practices and names. International and bilateral assistance
could perhaps contribute to financing translation into a number of languages. A
physician might be specially appointed by the ministry of health or the working
group to be responsible for the translation and publication. One need hardly
stress the importance of accuracy, since an error in translation or printing
could have serious consequences.

5.3 Once it has been adapted and translated, the national working guide should
be issued in a format which PHWs can use easily during their training and, later,
for reference and for continuing education. It should be able to stand up to the
hard conditions of community work, and it should also allow for new information to
be added. A loose-leaf format would permit new material to be prepared for later
training sessions, but it might be more expensive and less hard-wearing and there
is a serious risk that pages may be lost or new material not inserted.

The present WHO book is in three parts, of which only the first, the entitled
"Working Guide", is intended for PHWs. The second part, "Guidelines for Training"
is meant for trainers of PHWs, and the third, "Guidelines for Adaptation", is of
concern to health administrators and trainers. It seems logical that only the
first part should be given to PHWs, and that it should therefore be printed
separately from the two other parts. The annexes on medicines and techniques
should be included with Part I; but whether or not to include the anatomical
diagrams should be discussed.

The first edition of the national working guide - adapted as necessary - might
be printed cheaply for field testing. Feedback from field testing would make it
possible to correct errors, modify the text or its presentation, and add important
comments or material. This would improve the second edition, make it more valuable
and justify its wide distribution.